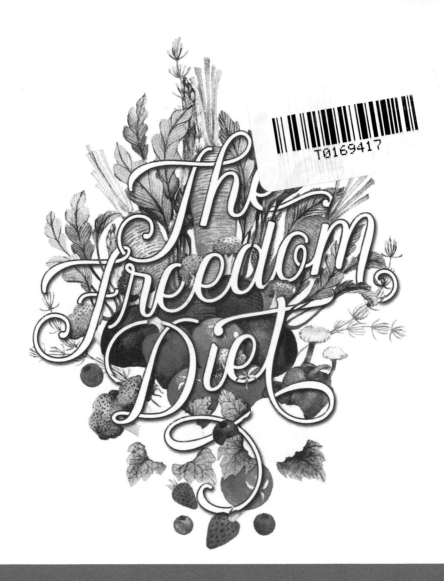

COOKBOOK

LOWER BLOOD SUGAR, LOSE WEIGHT, AND

CHANGE YOUR LIFE IN 60 DAYS

JESSICA BLACK, N.D.

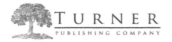

TURNER
PUBLISHING COMPANY

Turner Publishing Company

424 Church Street • Suite 2240 • Nashville, Tennessee 37219

445 Park Avenue • 9th Floor • New York, New York 10022

www.turnerpublishing.com

Cover design: Patrick Cabral and Maddie Cothren
Book design: Mallory Collins

Library of Congress Cataloging-in-Publication Data

Names: Black, Jessica, author.
Title: The freedom diet cookbook : lower blood sugar, lose weight and change
  your life in 60 days / by Jessica Black.
Description: Nashville, Tennessee : Turner Publishing Company, [2016] |
  Includes bibliographical references and index.
Identifiers: LCCN 2015034741 | ISBN 9781681621166 (pbk. : alk. paper)
Subjects: LCSH: Diet therapy--Popular works. | Nutrition--Recipes--Popular
  works. | Self-care, Health--Popular works. | Food preferences. | Weight
  loss--Popular works. | Cookbooks. lcgft
Classification: LCC RA784 .B5514 2016 | DDC 641.5/635--dc23
LC record available at http://lccn.loc.gov/2015034741

10 9 8 7 6 5 4 3 2 1

CONTENTS

CHAPTER 2: SNACKS, SIDES, APPETIZERS, AND CONDIMENTS

CHAPTER 3: SALADS

CHAPTER 4: SOUPS

CHAPTER 5: ENTREES

CHAPTER 6: BEVERAGES

CHAPTER 7: DESSERTS

PREFACE

It is not always easy to maintain health. In fact, it takes continual persistence to treat or prevent chronic illness through diet and lifestyle. From exercise to diet to keeping your mental and emotional sides happy, changing your health takes effort.

I like to use the analogy of a boat traveling downstream. When things are going in the wrong direction and your health is getting worse, you are simply drifting downstream toward death. The first phase of getting better involves reversing the direction of your "boat." These initial efforts are the hardest because you are not used to the new habits and the required lifestyle changes. Once the boat is turned around, it will always be traveling upstream. If you have ever paddled a kayak you understand how much more difficult it is to go upstream than down. Just as it is easier to allow a boat to passively drift downstream, it is very easy for us to be complacent and accept the fact that we don't feel as good as we once did, that our energy is lower and we don't have the same zest for life. It is also easy for us to allow new diagnoses to creep in as long as we don't experience obvious symptoms, and then to believe that we don't need to make any efforts to change.

Change is hard. When you first start a new diet or lifestyle habit, it can be challenging to maintain. You must remember that turning the boat around is the hardest part, but once you have it cruising upstream, continuing in that direction will be less difficult. If you successfully use the Freedom Diet to help you lose weight, feel better, or improve your blood sugar, then it is up to you to remember the importance of your newly improved health and to continually strive to maintain it. After you have completed the 60-day challenge outlined in the book *The Freedom Diet*, I challenge you to commit to a future of making the effort required to keep your health on track.

Although I practice naturopathic medicine and make use of hundreds of different remedies, medicines, and therapies, my favorites by far are lifestyle changes, and I'll tell you why. You can take a pharmaceutical medicine or a natural medicine to treat a symptom, but if you don't do anything to truly change the disease process, as soon as that medicine is no longer at your disposal, your symptoms will return and you'll risk going back to the same state of health you were in before taking the medicine. In that scenario, the medicines haven't done much to change your health. Early in my practice, I decided that along with whatever medicines I prescribed, I would always ensure that my patients were doing something for themselves to change their underlying health picture. I adopted the goal of helping my patients embrace new health habits that would create new patterns in their bodies and for their futures.

The strongest changes you can make for your health don't involve taking medicines or finding the newest supplement for your ailment; rather, they come from improving your habits of diet and exercise, availing yourself of clean water and clean air, paying attention to your mental and emotional health, and maintaining happiness.

Let food be thy medicine and medicine be thy food.

— Hippocrates

ACKNOWLEDGMENTS

I am so thankful to my family for supporting me through the process of working hard to simultaneously write *The Freedom Diet* and this recipe book. Thank you to my eldest daughter, Sadie, for personally testing many of these recipes while I tested other ones or continued writing.

I also want to thank my younger daughter and my husband for being honest reviewers of the recipes. I always love to hear sounds of delight as my family members eat their meals.

To my mom, who never used any measuring cups or measuring spoons, thank you for teaching me how to improvise and how to cook and bake creatively. I feel like I have a strong enough foundation in the kitchen that I can whip up meals seemingly out of nothing, and I want to thank you for teaching me that.

INTRODUCTION

The Freedom Diet is a way to transform your life for the better. I have been prescribing this diet for years in my practice, and I have seen amazing health transitions. In fact, I have advocated dietary changes to my patients for my entire time in practice because I feel that a good diet lays the best foundation possible for medicines and other therapies to work more effectively.

Cleaning up your diet is one of the most important things you can do for your health. The state of our society's health is deteriorating, and one major cause is the dietary choices that many people make, unfortunately from the time they're very young. The prevalence of diabetes and obesity in our country is depressing. Sugar is consumed by children and teenagers in great quantities. Fried foods, processed foods, foods with additives, and other detrimental foods are widespread throughout the world. The number-one cause of death in the world is heart disease, and numerous studies support the idea that diet and lifestyle changes can be just as or more effective than pharmaceutical medications targeted to reducing cardiovascular risk. When you take a pharmaceutical medication, it has only one targeted effect. But when you start exercising regularly and consuming healthy foods, you not only reduce cardiovascular risk; you also experience body-wide benefits.

The Freedom Diet was designed as an aggressive sixty-day plan to reduce blood sugar and insulin resistance. As I prescribed it to more people, I found the benefits to be tremendous. I started recommending it to a broader population and noticed that most people benefited.

The Freedom Diet helps people lose weight, feel better, decrease their risk for chronic disease, reduce blood sugar, and often reduce pain. If you strictly stick to the plan for sixty days, you will see benefits. To enjoy the full advantage the program has to offer, especially if you are trying to reverse diabetes or bring down your blood sugar levels, then also consider trying the Glucose Freedom Supplement that is part of the complete sixty-day plan. You can read more about the supplement plan in the accompanying book *The Freedom Diet*, or at my website, www.drjessicablack.com.

What should you do after you have completed the sixty-day challenge? Simply said, maintain the diet as well as you can. You can either stick with the Freedom Diet for longer, or you can transition into the Anti-Inflammation Diet (the topic of two of my earlier books), which allows a larger range of foods to choose from. Whatever you choose, remember to commit to it for the rest of your life (at least most of the time). If you find that you've had a day when you didn't do well, simply pick up the next day and do better. Don't let bad habits creep back in, and if they do, recognize them and do something about it. Surround yourself with other people interested in changing their health through better diet, and discuss and exchange recipes with them. Find an exercise buddy, and commit to working out or walking together a few days per week. These strategies can help keep you engaged while you're on your new path to improved health and lifestyle habits.

BE PREPARED AND DON'T BE AFRAID

Success is no accident. It is hard work, perseverance,
learning, studying, sacrifice, and most of all, love
of what you are doing or learning to do.
— PELE

Here are a few hints to help you with the Freedom Diet. Initially it can be really hard to give up sweets; therefore, it is most important to strictly avoid all sugar for at least the first thirty days. After that, your sugar cravings will most likely decrease considerably. If you keep eating sugar, then you may continue to be plagued with cravings .

I love food and food preparation. You might find me geeking out in the kitchen store over the best new slicer or a unique new pan, but I try to keep my supplies simple. I like having a good knife and cutting board and a few nice pans. I use cast iron because I inherited them from my husband's grandmother, and they are well-cured and relatively nonstick. I also have a cast-iron wok that I use occasionally.

I can guarantee that anyone who eats eight cups of vegetables per day for a few weeks will experience some sort of improvement in their health. The main problem people encounter when first boosting their vegetable intake is that their digestion may not be ready for the change, causing them to feel awfully gassy. The simple solution is to steam all your vegetables (except salad greens), which will aid your digestion.

You will find that the recipes offer easy suggestions to help you see that cooking can be rather quick and uncomplicated, especially when you use simple ingredients.

Taking lunches and snacks along with you when you leave the house prevents you from getting lost in the American wasteland of fast food if you become urgently hungry. Resisting the temptations of sweets and treats at work takes willpower and backbone. Understanding creates willpower—understanding the risks involved in making poor food choices and the risk inflammation and elevated blood sugar pose to your long-term health, and understanding how great it feels to enjoy vibrant health and well-being.

Finally, do the best you can, and don't beat yourself up along the way. If you make a mistake, pull yourself up, brush yourself off, and keep going. Know that with any change, you are bound to make mistakes.

Don't be afraid to fail. Behind every success often lie a significant number of failures. Be creative. Don't think you have to follow the recipes or the lifestyle plan verbatim. Make them your own thing. Create your own meals from the ideas presented in this book, and learn to season foods in your own unique way. Experiment a lot! Your experiments may result in the occasional funny moment in your kitchen or at the dinner table with your family, but they will also force you to learn and improve your skills.

NAVIGATING FOOD CHOICES

Food is prepared in many ways. Sometimes the method of food preparation can interfere with the food's quality and nutrient content. Below are my suggestions for choosing foods that are as natural and nutrient-dense as possible. The main goal with this food plan is to get back to our roots. That means greatly reducing or eliminating consumption of artificial additives, chemicals, preservatives, and unnatural substances, many of which have been linked to cancer and other illnesses.

- *Filter your drinking and cooking water.* Consider this a golden rule in your kitchen and for your family. Plain tap water simply contains too many chemicals that can affect your health, such as heavy metals, hormones, residues from chemicals used in treatment facilities, and farming chemicals. Furthermore, the balance of minerals in your water may be off. A filter can help remove unwanted chemicals and correct imbalances. Many different types of water filters are available; spend some time researching them before purchasing one. You can begin with a simple system, like a Brita pitcher, which utilizes a carbon filter, but for the long term consider going with a more advanced filtration system for your entire home.

- *Organic meat is best.* Organic meat is free of toxic chemicals. If you can't always find organic meat, then look for hormone-free meat. Organic meat usually comes from animals that have been grass fed or, in the case of poultry, have been given feed free of additives such as antibiotics. Grass-fed animal proteins are better than proteins from grain-fed animals. Cattle and buffalo were meant to graze on grass, and that is what they do for most of their lives. Most commercially raised cattle will graze on grass but will be finished off in the last months of their lives with grains such as corn to increase their weight and fat content. The meat taste we have grown to love as Americans comes from this extra fat content. Grass-fed animals are leaner; they have ⅓ to ½ the fat of grain-fed animals of the same size. The meat from grass-fed animals is higher in good nutrients: Beef from a grass-fed cow has three times the vitamin E content and is higher in omega-3 fatty acids, providing a better omega-3 to omega-6 ratio, than beef from a grain-fed cow. Grass-fed beef also has a higher content of conjugated linoleic acid (CLA), a lesser-known but important group of polyunsaturated fatty acids found in beef, lamb, and dairy products. The less our farming practices adhere to an animal's natural growth and development patterns, the greater the risk of something going wrong, such as the meat being contaminated or the animal getting sick. It is also important to avoid meat from animals that have been fed antibiotics or hormones or have spent time around pesticides. Hormones fed to animals are used to increase their growth, but they are detrimental to health. Many of the common cancers, such as prostate, breast, and ovarian cancers, are often directly related to excess hormone influence.

- *Whenever possible, choose organic vegetables and fruits.* Produce is best purchased fresh and local. A few vegetables and fruits, such as peas and berries, may be purchased frozen for ease of use. Never buy canned vegetables and fruits, with the exception of canned tomatoes on rare occasions. If you are on a tight budget and organic produce seems out of reach cost-wise, be aware that there are a few fruits and vegetables that are more important to purchase organic because they are heavily sprayed with chemicals when grown following conventional methods. A comprehensive list of both the cleanest and the most contaminated fruits and vegetables can be found at the website of the Environmental Working Group: www.ewg.org/foodnews/summary.

- *Use Real Salt over other types of sea salt or table salt.* Many table salts contain added anticaking agents or dextrose, which is a potato sugar. Other types of sea salt are sometimes more processed and may not offer the variety of minerals that Real Salt does. Real Salt brand sea salt comes from Redmond, Utah, and has a distinct, rich taste. Its off-white color comes from the many trace minerals (as many as sixty different ones) that are present in the salt. Himalayan or Celtic salts are also acceptable, but I prefer using a salt local to our region rather than from other parts of the world.

- *Buy fresh foods over canned.* Exceptions to this guideline include coconut milk, canned wild-caught salmon, and beans (occasionally) when you are in a pinch and haven't soaked any.

- *Purchase wild-caught fish instead of farm-raised.* Wild fish contains significantly higher levels of omega-3 fatty acids, the important fats that help our bodies ward off cancer and other inflammatory illnesses. They are also extremely important in supporting brain function and helping maintain memory and cognitive ability into older age. Farmed fish such as salmon often contains dyes to make it appear rich in omega-3 fatty acids.

- *Avoid processed foods as much as possible.* Chips, boxed foods, prepared meals, cold cuts, hot dogs, frozen pizzas, frozen snacks, SpaghettiOs, and prepared macaroni and cheese are just some examples of processed foods that should be avoided.

FOOD ITEMS TO KEEP ON HAND/SHOPPING LIST

Below is a list of some helpful items to keep in your kitchen. Having these groceries on hand can minimize your trips to the store when you're planning a meal and will make it easier to throw together healthy dinners spontaneously. A meal of beans and rice is an easy staple you can prepare in a pinch, even if you haven't been able to go grocery shopping.

- dried grains and legumes: quinoa, lentils, white beans, garbanzo beans
- canned goods: salmon, beans, coconut milk
- dried spices: cinnamon, ginger, basil, garlic powder, onion powder, mustard powder, cumin, turmeric, nutmeg, peppercorns or fresh-ground pepper, Real Salt
- other dried goods: unsweetened coconut, sunflower seeds, pumpkin seeds, hemp seeds, chia seeds, flaxseeds
- fresh vegetables in season, including salad greens
- fresh berries
- frozen goods: homemade broths, berries for smoothies
- condiments: gluten-free tamari sauce, mustard with no added sugar, homemade mayonnaise

- vinegars: apple cider vinegar, red wine vinegar, white vinegar, others as desired
- fresh herbs and spices: garlic, onions, ginger, parsley
- fats and oils: organic butter, coconut oil, olive oil
- milk and eggs: unsweetened almond milk, unsweetened hemp milk, organic eggs
- specifics for the recipes you want to prepare during the week

MAKING HEALTHY EATING EASIER

It is important to reduce kitchen time and make your kitchen and yourself more efficient. This task is not always easy, especially with our busy lifestyles involving work, kids in sports, and other commitments. Here are a few tips for reducing kitchen time.

Food Preparation
- Prechop vegetables you know you will be using during the week.
- Prechop garlic and onions, and keep them refrigerated in airtight containers.
- Prepare everything for dinner when you are making lunch so that dinner is much easier to get on the table.
- Make stocks and broths ahead of time, and store them in small quantities in the freezer.
- Make large batches of soup so you have extra to freeze for a later date.
- Prepare extra servings when you're cooking dinner so you have leftovers for lunch the next day.
- Do not microwave food. If you microwave at all, do so sparingly because the process destroys important nutrients.

Equipment

- Small food chopper.
- Coffee grinder or spice grinder (for grinding nuts and seeds).
- Blender or Vitamix. A Vitamix is an extremely high-powered blender that can handle a full range of tasks, from making a smoothie to grinding nuts and seeds to making flours. If you have a Vitamix, then you generally won't need a coffee grinder or food chopper.
- Food processor. Superior to the Vitamix for grating a large quantity of an ingredient such as zucchini or another vegetable, especially if you don't want your vegetables to be cut too fine.
- Mandoline. A mandoline is a professional food slicer that is great for quickly slicing onions, carrots, cabbage, etc. I no longer use my food processor unless I need it for large batches of grated zucchini, for example. I love the mandoline because it is easy to use for any amount of vegetables, works very quickly, and is easy to clean. Mandolines can be purchased online or in a kitchen store.
- Nonaluminum sauté pans and ovenware.
- Parchment paper. Parchment paper has saved me hundreds of hours of cleaning time. You can line any baking pan with parchment paper for a nearly hassle-free cleanup.

Cooking Tips

- Use easy steaming procedures for simple vegetable side dishes topped with a small amount of your favorite sauce. You can use an inexpensive basket-style steamer, or just put ½ inch of filtered water in a saucepan, add chopped vegetables, and cook over medium heat. With either method, steam until the vegetables have a bright color but are still crunchy-tender. You may need to add more water if it evaporates during steaming. Additionally, you can save the water that you steamed your vegetables in and add it to a smoothie or cook lentils in it so that you still obtain the nutrients that have leached into the water.

- Learn to improvise! Don't think you always need a recipe. The more you cook, the more you will learn to guess what you need, and the more you will learn about how seasonings blend together. You'll get better at substituting when you don't have the exact ingredient. Don't be afraid to experiment with new ingredients.
- Make extra servings of lentils or beans when preparing a meal, and freeze the extra in airtight containers. It is handy to be able to thaw some frozen lentils and add them to a salad or other meal to boost the protein content.
- Eat raw one night per week. This can be an easy meal of cut-up veggies, fruits, and dips. Often, we will throw veggies and fruit into the blender with water and have a green drink for the evening. This feels very refreshing and healthy. Make sure you are able to tolerate raw foods before incorporating "Raw Night" into your household.

Organization and Preparation

- Keep your pantry, refrigerator, and spice area well organized.
- Make lists when you run out of items that you need from the store.
- Plan meals before you grocery shop.
- Have "go to" meals that are easy and quick, but still nutritious and healthy. This helps to reduce unhealthy snacking.
- Have ideas for healthy snacks, and avoid buying snacks that you will feel guilty about eating.
- Clean the kitchen as you prepare meals. Utilize the natural gaps

in time that occur during cooking to wash the dishes and utensils you have used and no longer need. That way, many of your dishes are already rinsed and placed in the dishwasher before your meal is ready to eat.

- Pack your lunches, and take snacks with you everywhere you go. Don't rely on finding food while you're out. Most of the time you won't be able to find much that's healthy. Carrying snacks will also keep you and your children happier by helping you avoid blood sugar crashes and the resulting moodiness.

Food Attitude

- Have fun when you go shopping. Take the whole family so that you all participate in choosing foods. Think about foods and cooking from a new perspective. Don't fight the change; accept and appreciate it for what it will bring to you and your family.
- Get the children involved. Have them pick out a new vegetable at the store, and then go home and research how to cook it.
- Grow a garden so that you have control over what you grow and so that you can enjoy eating from the crop you harvest. Even if you don't have garden space, many plants can be grown on a sunny patio.

SAMPLE FIVE-DAY HABIT CHART

	Monday	Tuesday	Wednesday	Thursday	Friday
Cardio Exercise	Walking or jogging	Zumba	Yoga	Walking or jogging	Elliptical or treadmill
Weight training	Light to moderate weights	None	Light to moderate weights	None	Light to moderate weights
Water	½ body weight in oz	½ body weight in oz	½ body weight in oz	½ body weight in oz	½ body weight in oz
Supplements	Glucose Freedom 4 capsules	Glucose Freedom 4 capsules	Glucose Freedom 4 capsules	Glucose Freedom 4 capsules	Glucose Freedom 4 capsules
Meditation	5 minutes*	5 minutes	5 minutes	5 minutes	5 minutes
Affirmations	Say out loud 3 sentences**	Say out loud 3 sentences	Say out loud 3 sentences	Say out loud 3 sentences	Say out loud 3 sentences
Breakfast*	Poached Eggs and Greens with Hollandaise	Chia Flax Pudding with green drink	Sautéed Zucchini with Eggs and Avocado	Hard-boiled egg with green salad	Squash Pancakes
Snack	Pumpkin seeds	Celery with sunflower butter	Avocado with lemon and tamari	Sunflower seeds	Spicy Seed Crackers
Lunch	Sausage Soup and salad	Romaine Greek Salad	Easy Salmon Salad	Romaine Sandwich with Roasted Squash Rings	Kale Caesar Salad
Fiber Supplement	Taken with 12 oz filtered water and very small snack if desired	Taken with 12 oz filtered water and very small snack if desired	Taken with 12 oz filtered water and very small snack if desired	Taken with 12 oz filtered water and very small snack if desired	Taken with 12 oz filtered water and very small snack if desired
Supplements	Glucose Freedom 4 capsules	Glucose Freedom 4 capsules	Glucose Freedom 4 capsules	Glucose Freedom 4 capsules	Glucose Freedom 4 capsules
Dinner	Jicama Fish Tacos	Collard Green Roll-Ups	Spaghetti Squash with Meat sauce	Red Lentil Soup and salad	Green Curry
Affirmations	Say affirmations again or spend a few minutes visualizing yourself healthy	Say affirmations again or spend a few minutes visualizing yourself healthy	Say affirmations again or spend a few minutes visualizing yourself healthy	Say affirmations again or spend a few minutes visualizing yourself healthy	Say affirmations again or spend a few minutes visualizing yourself healthy
Sleep	Get at least 8 hours of sleep	Get at least 8 hours of sleep	Get at least 8 hours of sleep	Get at least 8 hours of sleep	Get at least 8 hours of sleep
Stay motivated	Keep at it	You're doing great	It's worth it	Health is a reward	Smile and stick with it

*Over time, you should be able to increase the number of minutes you meditate per day. Start with 5 minutes as a manageable goal; each week, add 5 minutes per day until you have reached 10–20 minutes, or whatever you are willing to spare.

**Sample sentences are noted in the chapter titled "Habits to Include."

***If you are not a breakfast person, simply make a green drink with 1 raw egg for protein, and slowly sip it throughout the morning.

MEASUREMENT CONVERSION CHARTS

Liquid Measures

1 cup = 8 fluid ounces = 250 ml

1 tablespoon = ½ fluid ounce = 16 ml

1 teaspoon = ⅙ fluid ounce = 5⅓ ml

16 tablespoons = 1 cup

3 teaspoons = 1 tablespoon

Egg Sizes

(Large is the US standard for cooking.)

1 egg = 1.5 fluid ounces = 1.75 ounces without shell = 50 grams
without shell

1 egg white = 2 tablespoons = 32 milliliters = 30 grams

1 egg yolk = 1 tablespoon = 16 milliliters = 20 grams

Solid Fats (Butter, Coconut Oil)

8 tablespoons = 4 ounces = ¼ pound = 115 grams

butter: 1 stick = 8 tablespoons = 4 ounces = ¼ pound = 115 grams

Temperatures

250°F = 120°C = very low

200°F = 150°C = low

325°F = 165°C = moderately low

350°F = 180°C = moderate

375°F = 190°C = moderately hot

400°F = 200°C = hot

450°F = 230°C = very hot

500°F = 260°C = extremely hot; most broilers are set at this
temperature or above

Chapter 1

BREAKFASTS

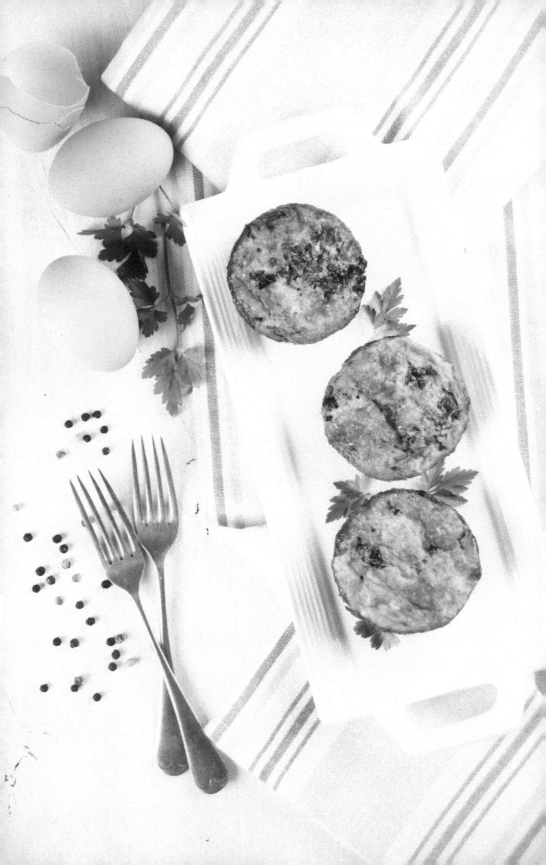

MINI QUICHE CUPS

INGREDIENTS

10 eggs

1 red bell pepper, minced

2 cups tightly packed raw spinach, chopped fine

1 cup shredded sharp cheddar cheese (omit if dairy intolerant)

¼ cup minced chives

½ teaspoon salt

½ teaspoon pepper

Grease two 6-cup muffin pans or one 12-cup muffin pan. Heat oven to 350°F. Beat the eggs together in a large bowl with a fork; add remaining ingredients and combine. Evenly pour egg mixture among the 12 muffin cups. Bake for 15 to 20 minutes or until a toothpick inserted into the center of one comes out clean.

Macronutrients		
Kilocalories	102.559	kcal
Protein	7.780	g
Carbohydrate	1.304	g
Fat, Total	7.207	g
Alcohol	0.000	g
Cholesterol	164.605	mg
Saturated Fat	3.135	g
Monounsaturated Fat	2.320	g
Polyunsaturated Fat	0.950	g
Trans Fatty Acid	0.016	g
Dietary Fiber, Total	0.365	g
Sugar, Total	0.637	g
Percentage of Kcals		
Protein	30.8%	
Carbohydrate	5.2%	
Fat, total	64.1%	
Alcohol	0.0%	
Vitamins & Minerals		
Sodium	221.099	mg
Potassium	117.624	mg
Vitamin A (RE)	178.129	RE
Vitamin C	14.650	mg
Calcium	93.908	mg
Iron	0.948	mg
Vitamin D (ug)	0.890	µg
Vitamin E (mg)	0.472	mg
Thiamin	0.029	mg
Riboflavin	0.250	mg
Niacin	0.176	mg
Pyridoxine (Vitamin B6)	0.116	mg
Folate (Total)	37.358	µg
Cobalamin (Vitamin B12)	0.454	µg
Biotin	0.588	µg
Pantothenic Acid	0.723	mg
Vitamin K	27.299	µg
Phosphorus	132.787	mg
Magnesium	13.255	mg
Zinc	0.919	mg
Copper	0.046	mg
Manganese	0.086	mg
Selenium	15.530	µg
Chromium	0.001	mg
Molybdenum	1.683	µg

Serves 12.

Recipe Tidbit:

Making these mini quiches ahead of time can provide you with a very simple protein snack. They can even be eaten cold. If you are dairy intolerant, simply omit the cheese and add 2 more eggs to evenly fill the 12 muffin cups. You can get very creative with the recipe by adding ingredients such as cooked sausage, other vegetables, onions, garlic, and any spices you desire (see the recipe on page 34 for one suggested variation).

AVOCADO EGGS

INGREDIENTS

1 medium to large ripe avocado
2 small to medium eggs

Heat oven to 425°F. Leaving the rind intact, gently cut the avocado in half lengthwise and remove the pit. Make a small cut on the rind side of each avocado half in order to prevent them from tilting when baking. Carve some of the flesh out of each avocado half to make a hole big enough for the egg, and place each half flesh side up in a baking dish. You can use a soufflé dish or ramekin. Crack two eggs into a separate bowl, and spoon a yolk into each avocado half. Fill the avocados to the top with the remaining egg white, top with salt and pepper, and transfer to oven. Bake for 10 to 15 minutes or until the yolk is cooked to your taste.

Serves 2.

Macronutrients		
Kilocalories	183.124	kcal
Protein	7.590	g
Carbohydrate	6.135	g
Fat, Total	15.055	g
Alcohol	0.000	g
Cholesterol	186.000	mg
Saturated Fat	2.984	g
Monounsaturated Fat	8.379	g
Polyunsaturated Fat	2.169	g
Trans Fatty Acid	0.019	g
Dietary Fiber, Total	4.545	g
Sugar, Total	0.386	g

Percentage of Kcals	
Protein	15.9%
Carbohydrate	12.9%
Fat, total	71.2%
Alcohol	0.0%

Vitamins & Minerals		
Sodium	76.347	mg
Potassium	407.883	mg
Vitamin A (RE)	90.833	RE
Vitamin C	5.882	mg
Calcium	36.689	mg
Iron	1.283	mg
Vitamin D (ug)	1.000	µg
Vitamin E (mg)	0.526	mg
Thiamin	0.070	mg
Riboflavin	0.324	mg
Niacin	1.315	mg
Pyridoxine (Vitamin B6)	0.277	mg
Folate (Total)	82.988	µg
Cobalamin (Vitamin B12)	0.445	µg
Pantothenic Acid	1.744	mg
Vitamin K	14.187	µg
Phosphorus	135.094	mg
Magnesium	25.384	mg
Zinc	1.100	mg
Copper	0.150	mg
Manganese	0.114	mg
Selenium	15.617	µg

Recipe Tidbit:

Avocados are such an amazing food. They can be used for savory or sweet dishes, but most of the time we eat them cold. I predict you will enjoy this warm variation. It is a very simple breakfast to prepare. You can top the avocado eggs with anything you would like before or after baking. For a delicious addition, top them with fresh salsa and crumbled cotija (a Mexican cheese) as they come out of the oven.

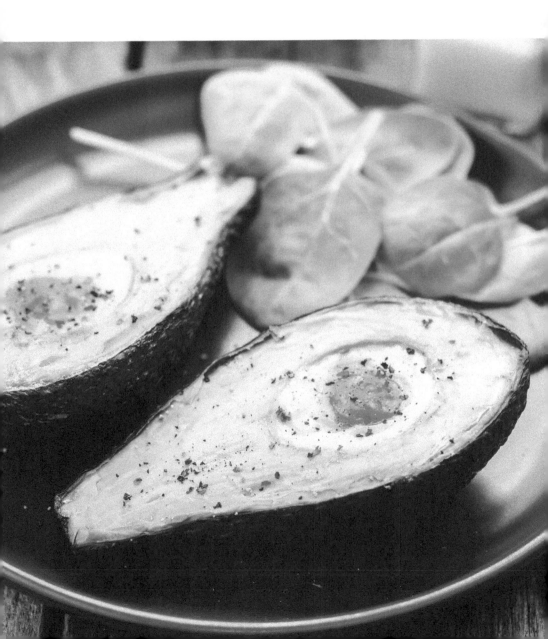

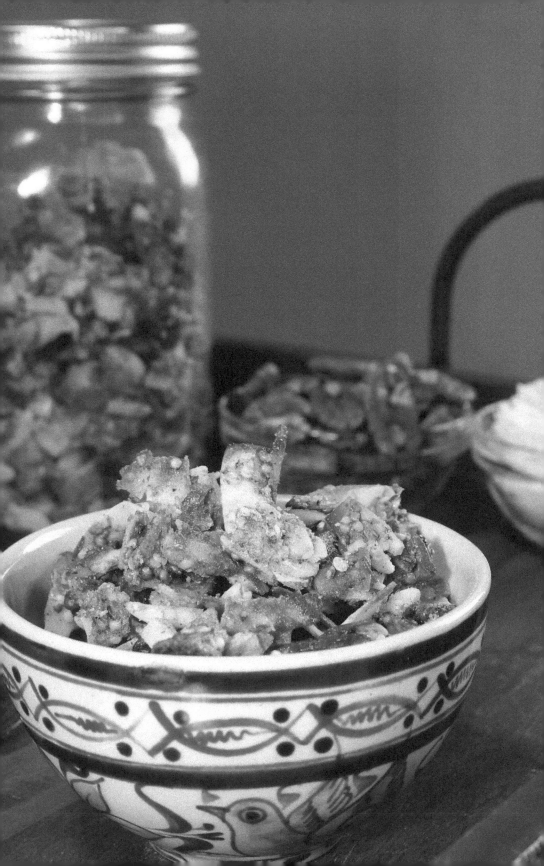

COCONUT NUTTY GRANOLA

INGREDIENTS

1½ cups flaked unsweetened
   coconut

1 cup slivered almonds

½ cup hemp seeds

½ cup pecans

1 teaspoon cinnamon

½ teaspoon dried ginger

½ teaspoon nutmeg

2 large eggs or 3 small eggs, lightly
   beaten with a fork

1 teaspoon vanilla extract

Macronutrients		
Kilocalories	317.069	kcal
Protein	10.434	g
Carbohydrate	9.817	g
Fat, Total	28.332	g
Alcohol	0.206	g
Cholesterol	53.143	mg
Saturated Fat	9.731	g
Monounsaturated Fat	8.574	g
Polyunsaturated Fat	3.860	g
Trans Fatty Acid	0.008	g
Dietary Fiber, Total	5.416	g
Sugar, Total	1.982	g

Percentage of Kcals	
Protein	12.4%
Carbohydrate	11.6%
Fat, total	75.6%
Alcohol	0.4%

Vitamins & Minerals		
Sodium	24.872	mg
Potassium	289.278	mg
Vitamin A (RE)	23.744	RE
Vitamin C	0.104	mg
Calcium	58.747	mg
Iron	2.621	mg
Vitamin D (ug)	0.286	µg
Vitamin E (mg)	0.668	mg
Thiamin	0.089	mg
Riboflavin	0.252	mg
Niacin	0.681	mg
Pyridoxine (Vitamin B6)	0.064	mg
Folate (Total)	15.372	µg
Cobalamin (Vitamin B12)	0.127	µg
Biotin	4.086	µg
Pantothenic Acid	0.361	mg
Vitamin K	0.419	µg
Phosphorus	124.861	mg
Magnesium	131.338	mg
Zinc	1.033	mg
Copper	0.267	mg
Manganese	1.940	mg
Selenium	5.399	µg

Preheat oven to 350°F. Thoroughly mix together all dry ingredients. Add the eggs and vanilla, and combine until uniform. Spread on a baking sheet and bake until the mixture has browned, about 15 to 20 minutes. Every 5 minutes while baking, take the mixture out of the oven and stir. Remove from oven, allow to cool, and store in airtight container. Serve with unsweetened almond milk topped with berries of your choice.

Serves 7.

SPINACH AND SALMON MINI QUICHE CUPS

INGREDIENTS

12 eggs

2 cups tightly packed raw spinach, chopped fine

1 5-ounce can boneless, skinless wild-caught salmon

¼ minced cup chives

2 tablespoons mayonnaise

½ teaspoon salt

½ teaspoon pepper

½ teaspoon dill

Grease two 6-cup muffin pans or one 12-cup muffin pan. Heat oven to 350°F. Beat the eggs together in a large bowl with a fork; add remaining ingredients and combine. Evenly pour egg mixture among the 12 muffin cups. Bake for 15 to 20 minutes or until a toothpick inserted into the center comes out clean.

Serves 12.

Macronutrients		
Kilocalories	107.831	kcal
Protein	9.713	g
Carbohydrate	0.655	g
Fat, Total	7.187	g
Alcohol	0.000	g
Cholesterol	195.117	mg
Saturated Fat	1.947	g
Monounsaturated Fat	2.489	g
Polyunsaturated Fat	2.185	g
Trans Fatty Acid	0.023	g
Dietary Fiber, Total	0.157	g
Sugar, Total	0.238	g

Percentage of Kcals	
Protein	36.6%
Carbohydrate	2.5%
Fat, total	60.9%
Alcohol	0.0%

Vitamins & Minerals		
Sodium	232.570	mg
Potassium	145.266	mg
Vitamin A (RE)	140.286	RE
Vitamin C	1.993	mg
Calcium	37.825	mg
Iron	1.266	mg
Vitamin D (ug)	1.005	µg
Vitamin E (mg)	0.526	mg
Thiamin	0.027	mg
Riboflavin	0.264	mg
Niacin	1.274	mg
Pyridoxine (Vitamin B6)	0.109	mg
Folate (Total)	35.218	µg
Cobalamin (Vitamin B12)	1.028	µg
Biotin	0.620	µg
Pantothenic Acid	0.864	mg
Vitamin K	30.314	µg
Phosphorus	133.368	mg
Magnesium	14.329	mg
Zinc	0.760	mg
Copper	0.063	mg
Manganese	0.079	mg
Selenium	20.227	µg
Chromium	0.001	mg
Molybdenum	1.250	µg

PEACH EGGNOG

INGREDIENTS

4 eggs

1 cup coconut milk

1 cup unsweetened almond milk

½ cup frozen peaches

1 teaspoon vanilla extract

½ teaspoon nutmeg

½ teaspoon cinnamon

½ teaspoon cardamom

½ teaspoon xanthan gum (optional)

Combine all ingredients in a high-powered blender and blend until smooth. Serve immediately.

Serves 2.

Macronutrients		
Kilocalories	513.747	kcal
Protein	19.916	g
Carbohydrate	20.670	g
Fat, Total	40.609	g
Alcohol	0.722	g
Cholesterol	372.000	mg
Saturated Fat	28.892	g
Monounsaturated Fat	5.398	g
Polyunsaturated Fat	3.479	g
Trans Fatty Acid	0.038	g
Dietary Fiber, Total	5.953	g
Sugar, Total	13.506	g
Percentage of Kcals		
Protein	15.0%	
Carbohydrate	15.5%	
Fat, total	68.6%	
Alcohol	0.9%	
Vitamins & Minerals		
Sodium	175.422	mg
Potassium	685.474	mg
Vitamin A (RE)	181.181	RE
Vitamin C	64.864	mg
Calcium	104.352	mg
Iron	4.766	mg
Vitamin D (ug)	2.000	µg
Vitamin E (mg)	1.381	mg
Thiamin	0.081	mg
Riboflavin	0.479	mg
Niacin	1.362	mg
Pyridoxine (Vitamin B6)	0.223	mg
Folate (Total)	68.243	µg
Cobalamin (Vitamin B12)	0.890	µg
Pantothenic Acid	1.825	mg
Vitamin K	1.766	µg
Phosphorus	326.362	mg
Magnesium	61.765	mg
Zinc	2.181	mg
Copper	0.415	mg
Manganese	1.400	mg
Selenium	38.481	µg

Recipe Tidbit:

For thicker eggnog, add the xanthan gum gradually as a last step, making sure to blend thoroughly between additions to prevent clumping. Then allow the mixture to sit in the refrigerator for at least 30 minutes before consuming. If you need to save half of this mixture it should stay good in your refrigerator for two days.

Many individuals are nervous about eating raw eggs due to the chance of getting salmonella poisoning. This is a valid concern, but the risk of contracting salmonella from eggs is actually significantly low. The U.S. Department of Agriculture has indicated that salmonella incidence fell by 66 percent from 1998 to 2003. In the healthy individual, salmonella poisoning is a self-limiting disease that is quickly recovered from. Symptoms of salmonella poisoning include diarrhea, abdominal pain, nausea, vomiting, fever, and chills. It mostly strikes the elderly, infants, and those with compromised immune systems such as from cancer or HIV. The salmonella is acquired from fecal matter on the outside of the egg; therefore, make sure you wash eggs thoroughly before using them raw.

ZUCCHINI FRITTERS

INGREDIENTS

2 cups grated zucchini (about 3
medium zucchini)

1 teaspoon salt

½ onion, minced

2 cloves garlic, minced

1 tablespoon + 3 tablespoons
coconut oil

3 eggs, lightly beaten with a fork

1 tablespoon hemp seeds, ground

1 tablespoons chia seeds, ground

1 tablespoon pumpkin seeds,
ground

1 teaspoon dill

1 teaspoon black pepper

½ teaspoon baking powder

Macronutrients		
Kilocalories	114.022	kcal
Protein	3.793	g
Carbohydrate	2.945	g
Fat, Total	10.156	g
Alcohol	0.000	g
Cholesterol	69.750	mg
Saturated Fat	6.684	g
Monounsaturated Fat	1.290	g
Polyunsaturated Fat	1.034	g
Trans Fatty Acid	0.010	g
Dietary Fiber, Total	1.065	g
Sugar, Total	1.091	g

Percentage of Kcals	
Protein	12.8%
Carbohydrate	10.0%
Fat, total	77.2%
Alcohol	0.0%

Vitamins & Minerals		
Sodium	132.776	mg
Potassium	143.320	mg
Vitamin A (RE)	36.369	RE
Vitamin C	5.860	mg
Calcium	44.492	mg
Iron	0.848	mg
Vitamin D (ug)	0.375	µg
Vitamin E (mg)	0.197	mg
Thiamin	0.036	mg
Riboflavin	0.119	mg
Niacin	0.322	mg
Pyridoxine (Vitamin B6)	0.106	mg
Folate (Total)	18.239	µg
Cobalamin (Vitamin B12)	0.167	µg
Biotin	0.076	µg
Pantothenic Acid	0.382	mg
Vitamin K	1.854	µg
Phosphorus	81.774	mg
Magnesium	27.821	mg
Zinc	0.498	mg
Copper	0.063	mg
Manganese	0.319	mg
Selenium	6.759	µg
Chromium	0.003	mg

Combine zucchini with salt and toss. Allow to sit in a colander draining water for at least 10 minutes while preparing the other ingredients. Sauté the onion and garlic in 1 tablespoon coconut oil over medium heat for 3–5 minutes. Remove from heat and place in a large mixing bowl. Before using the zucchini, place a paper towel or cloth napkin over the top, and press down in the colander to drain any excess liquid. Then combine remaining ingredients in the mixing bowl.

Heat 3 tablespoons coconut oil in a large nonstick skillet over medium heat. Drop 2-tablespoon portions of the mixture into the pan, then use the back of a spoon to gently press the batter into 2-inch-wide fritters. Pan-fry until golden brown on both sides, 2-3 minutes per side. Transfer the fritters to a paper towel–lined plate. Repeat the process with the remaining batter. If the oil gets too dirty, feel free to discard it, add new oil, heat to temperature, and continue. Serve warm or at room temperature with lemon wedges.

Serves 8.

PORTABELLA EGGS BENEDICT

INGREDIENTS

1 portabella mushroom

1 tablespoon olive oil

1 cup raw spinach leaves, stems
   removed

2 eggs

4 cups water

1 tablespoon vinegar

pinch salt

Hollandaise Sauce:

1 egg yolk

1½ teaspoons warm water

1½ teaspoons fresh lemon juice

¼ teaspoons salt

¼ stick butter

Macronutrients		
Kilocalories	273.883	kcal
Protein	9.077	g
Carbohydrate	3.107	g
Fat, Total	25.493	g
Alcohol	0.000	g
Cholesterol	308.755	mg
Saturated Fat	10.637	g
Monounsaturated Fat	10.747	g
Polyunsaturated Fat	2.530	g
Trans Fatty Acid	0.486	g
Dietary Fiber, Total	0.887	g
Sugar, Total	1.450	g
Percentage of Kcals		
Protein	13.1%	
Carbohydrate	4.5%	
Fat, total	82.5%	
Alcohol	0.0%	
Vitamins & Minerals		
Sodium	472.985	mg
Potassium	322.344	mg
Vitamin A (RE)	364.928	RE
Vitamin C	5.690	mg
Calcium	59.070	mg
Iron	1.690	mg
Vitamin D (ug)	6.376	µg
Vitamin E (mg)	0.865	mg
Thiamin	0.073	mg
Riboflavin	0.362	mg
Niacin	2.045	mg
Pyridoxine (Vitamin B6)	0.208	mg
Folate (Total)	77.959	µg
Cobalamin (Vitamin B12)	0.656	µg
Biotin	4.821	µg
Pantothenic Acid	1.530	mg
Vitamin K	77.702	µg
Phosphorus	188.573	mg
Magnesium	23.032	mg
Zinc	1.158	mg
Copper	0.183	mg
Manganese	0.183	mg
Selenium	28.219	µg
Chromium	0.003	mg
Molybdenum	3.750	µg

First prepare the hollandaise sauce by beating together all ingredients except the butter. Warm the butter in a small saucepan over medium heat. Very slowly stir the warmed butter into the sauce mixture. Keep the sauce warm by covering it and keeping it on the stove top.

Slice the portabella mushroom lengthwise into two thin rounds; the result should be like two halves of an English muffin. Heat in olive oil over medium heat in a nonstick skillet for 2–3 minutes; flip and heat the other side for 2–3 minutes. Keep the mushroom halves covered in the warm skillet.

To poach eggs: Heat water and vinegar and pinch of salt to simmering in medium saucepan or skillet. Crack an egg and gently slide it into the water. Simmer very gently until whites are set and yolk is still somewhat soft, about 3 minutes. Gently remove from water with a slotted spoon.

Combine by layering all ingredients: Place the portabella slices on two plates, and top each with ½ cup spinach leaves, a poached egg, and ½ the hollandaise sauce. Serve immediately.

Serves 2.

SAUTÉED ZUCCHINI WITH EGGS AND AVOCADO

INGREDIENTS

1 medium zucchini, sliced
   about ¼ inch thick

1 tablespoon butter

1 egg

1 tablespoon olive oil

½ avocado, diced large

3 tablespoons minced parsley
   (remove stems before cutting)

salt and pepper to taste

Macronutrients		
Kilocalories	441.648	kcal
Protein	10.416	g
Carbohydrate	12.951	g
Fat, Total	40.789	g
Alcohol	0.000	g
Cholesterol	216.530	mg
Saturated Fat	12.322	g
Monounsaturated Fat	21.268	g
Polyunsaturated Fat	4.214	g
Trans Fatty Acid	0.484	g
Dietary Fiber, Total	6.876	g
Sugar, Total	5.390	g

Percentage of Kcals	
Protein	9.0%
Carbohydrate	11.2%
Fat, total	79.7%
Alcohol	0.0%

Vitamins & Minerals		
Sodium	189.903	mg
Potassium	985.308	mg
Vitamin A (RE)	236.501	RE
Vitamin C	55.928	mg
Calcium	87.116	mg
Iron	2.784	mg
Vitamin D (ug)	1.213	µg
Vitamin E (mg)	0.856	mg
Thiamin	0.169	mg
Riboflavin	0.524	mg
Niacin	2.353	mg
Pyridoxine (Vitamin B6)	0.607	mg
Folate (Total)	147.553	µg
Cobalamin (Vitamin B12)	0.469	µg
Pantothenic Acid	2.205	mg
Vitamin K	216.225	µg
Phosphorus	219.507	mg
Magnesium	66.573	mg
Zinc	1.860	mg
Copper	0.270	mg
Manganese	0.479	mg
Selenium	16.163	µg
Chromium	0.005	mg

Sauté zucchini in butter over medium heat in a nonstick skillet until warm and turning slightly brown, about 5 minutes. Remove from heat and cover. In another small skillet, warm olive oil to medium heat and crack egg into pan. Cook until the egg white turns white but the yolk is still soft. Flip and cook for another minute or until desired yolk hardness is reached. Place zucchini in a serving bowl, top with fried egg, and garnish with avocado and parsley. Add salt and pepper to taste.

Serves 1.

OLIVE AND BROCCOLI FRITTATA

INGREDIENTS

1 medium green bell pepper, chopped

1 medium red bell pepper, chopped

2 broccoli crowns, cut into bite-sized pieces

1 7-ounce jar or can of sliced green olives

8 large eggs, softly beaten

¼ cup unsweetened almond milk

2 cloves garlic, minced

1 shallot, minced

1 teaspoon dried oregano

1 tablespoon fresh rosemary, minced, or 1 teaspoon dried rosemary

1 cup grated Swiss cheese (optional)

Macronutrients		
Kilocalories	174.349	kcal
Protein	11.010	g
Carbohydrate	7.444	g
Fat, Total	11.893	g
Alcohol	0.000	g
Cholesterol	248.000	mg
Saturated Fat	2.834	g
Monounsaturated Fat	6.242	g
Polyunsaturated Fat	1.927	g
Trans Fatty Acid	0.025	g
Dietary Fiber, Total	2.263	g
Sugar, Total	1.929	g

Percentage of Kcals	
Protein	24.4%
Carbohydrate	16.5%
Fat, total	59.2%
Alcohol	0.0%

Vitamins & Minerals		
Sodium	625.255	mg
Potassium	364.425	mg
Vitamin A (RE)	191.995	RE
Vitamin C	85.902	mg
Calcium	90.634	mg
Iron	2.145	mg
Vitamin D (ug)	1.333	µg
Vitamin E (mg)	0.701	mg
Thiamin	0.090	mg
Riboflavin	0.390	mg
Niacin	0.747	mg
Pyridoxine (Vitamin B6)	0.324	mg
Folate (Total)	78.717	µg
Cobalamin (Vitamin B12)	0.593	µg
Pantothenic Acid	1.382	mg
Vitamin K	4.998	µg
Phosphorus	176.881	mg
Magnesium	29.559	mg
Zinc	1.167	mg
Copper	0.133	mg
Manganese	0.214	mg
Selenium	22.379	µg
Chromium	0.004	mg

Light the broiler. Quarter and seed the peppers, then broil them skin side up for 5–10 minutes until lightly browned. Remove peppers from the oven and place in a brown paper bag for 5 minutes. Remove them from the bag; remove the entire skin or at least remove all charred areas.

Reduce heat to 400°F. Generously grease a 9-inch round pan. Place broccoli, peppers, and olives in the pan, making sure to arrange them evenly. Beat remaining ingredients together and pour over vegetables. Bake for 35–40 minutes or until the center has set. Cool, slice into wedges, and serve warm. Serves 6.

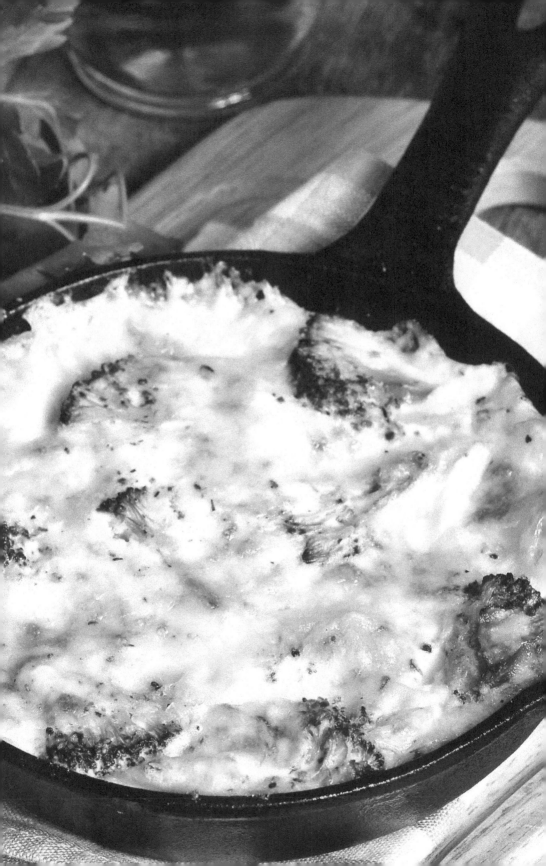

POACHED EGGS AND GREENS

INGREDIENTS

2 servings hollandaise sauce
(recipe on page 39)

2 eggs, poached (recipe on page 39)

1 cup arugula, chopped

1 cup kale, stems removed,
chopped

2 tablespoons minced fresh chives

First prepare the hollandaise sauce.
Keep the sauce warm by covering it
and keeping it on the stove top.

Next, poach the eggs.

Divide the greens between two
serving bowls. Top each serving
with a poached egg, cover with hollandaise sauce, and top with chives.
Serve immediately.

Serves 2.

Macronutrients		
Kilocalories	221.338	kcal
Protein	9.527	g
Carbohydrate	4.358	g
Fat, Total	18.917	g
Alcohol	0.000	g
Cholesterol	307.755	mg
Saturated Fat	9.708	g
Monounsaturated Fat	5.830	g
Polyunsaturated Fat	1.895	g
Trans Fatty Acid	0.484	g
Dietary Fiber, Total	1.452	g
Sugar, Total	1.355	g

Percentage of Kcals	
Protein	16.9%
Carbohydrate	7.7%
Fat, total	75.4%
Alcohol	0.0%

Vitamins & Minerals		
Sodium	550.240	mg
Potassium	295.962	mg
Vitamin A (RE)	587.476	RE
Vitamin C	44.918	mg
Calcium	111.903	mg
Iron	1.802	mg
Vitamin D (ug)	1.672	µg
Vitamin E (mg)	0.330	mg
Thiamin	0.076	mg
Riboflavin	0.299	mg
Niacin	0.428	mg
Pyridoxine (Vitamin B6)	0.206	mg
Folate (Total)	91.184	µg
Cobalamin (Vitamin B12)	0.545	µg
Biotin	13.770	µg
Pantothenic Acid	1.122	mg
Vitamin K	254.553	µg
Phosphorus	173.123	mg
Magnesium	28.687	mg
Zinc	1.107	mg
Copper	0.558	mg
Manganese	0.284	mg
Selenium	20.565	µg
Chromium	0.003	mg

BLUEBERRY SEED PANCAKES

INGREDIENTS

½ cup raw sunflower seeds,
   ground fine

½ cup raw pumpkin seeds, ground
   fine

½ teaspoon cinnamon

½ teaspoon baking powder

small pinch salt

¼ cup coconut oil, melted

5 eggs

½ cup blueberries

Macronutrients		
Kilocalories	832.143	kcal
Protein	31.926	g
Carbohydrate	11.490	g
Fat, Total	75.265	g
Alcohol	0.000	g
Cholesterol	465.000	mg
Saturated Fat	32.804	g
Monounsaturated Fat	14.930	g
Polyunsaturated Fat	20.282	g
Trans Fatty Acid	0.048	g
Dietary Fiber, Total	1.755	g
Sugar, Total	5.042	g
Percentage of Kcals		
Protein	15.0%	
Carbohydrate	5.4%	
Fat, total	79.6%	
Alcohol	0.0%	
Vitamins & Minerals		
Sodium	321.642	mg
Potassium	736.911	mg
Vitamin A (RE)	209.286	RE
Vitamin C	4.194	mg
Calcium	200.669	mg
Iron	8.180	mg
Vitamin D (ug)	2.500	µg
Vitamin E (mg)	15.257	mg
Thiamin	0.713	mg
Riboflavin	0.713	mg
Niacin	2.458	mg
Pyridoxine (Vitamin B6)	0.307	mg
Folate (Total)	81.004	µg
Cobalamin (Vitamin B12)	1.113	µg
Pantothenic Acid	1.963	mg
Vitamin K	7.687	µg
Phosphorus	855.244	mg
Magnesium	342.879	mg
Zinc	6.092	mg
Copper	1.409	mg
Manganese	1.049	mg
Selenium	56.071	µg

Combine the ground seeds, cinnamon, baking powder, salt, coconut oil, and eggs, and mix until clumps have dissolved. Add the blueberries, and stir just until mixture is uniform.

Heat a nonstick skillet or griddle pan over medium heat. Pour batter into pan, forming 3-inch circles. When pancakes begin to bubble, flip them and cook on the other side until lightly browned on both sides. Serve warm, topped with unsalted butter.

Serves 2.

Recipe Tidbit:

Instead of a pan manufactured with a nonstick coating, I use a very well cured cast-iron pan.

Note that these gluten-free pancakes won't bubble as much as regular wheat-flour pancakes. If you wait until the pancakes produce as many bubbles as you are used to before flipping them, you may burn them. After flipping them, I sometimes flip them back to the first side for a minute or so to ensure that they have cooked all the way through.

You can try using other berries in this recipe, or you can simply make the pancakes without berries.

PUMPKIN PANCAKES

INGREDIENTS

1 15-ounce can organic pumpkin

5 eggs

2 tablespoons coconut oil, melted

1 teaspoon vanilla extract

1 teaspoon cinnamon

1 teaspoon baking powder

½ teaspoon dried ginger

½ teaspoon nutmeg

½ teaspoon allspice

Macronutrients		
Kilocalories	205.275	kcal
Protein	2.487	g
Carbohydrate	19.967	g
Fat, Total	14.471	g
Alcohol	0.722	g
Cholesterol	0.000	mg
Saturated Fat	12.245	g
Monounsaturated Fat	0.894	g
Polyunsaturated Fat	0.295	g
Trans Fatty Acid	0.000	g
Dietary Fiber, Total	7.062	g
Sugar, Total	7.339	g
Percentage of Kcals		
Protein	4.4%	
Carbohydrate	35.5%	
Fat, total	57.9%	
Alcohol	2.2%	
Vitamins & Minerals		
Sodium	255.310	mg
Potassium	459.348	mg
Vitamin A (RE)	3309.743	RE
Vitamin C	9.180	mg
Calcium	206.848	mg
Iron	3.452	mg
Vitamin D (ug)	0.000	µg
Thiamin	0.054	mg
Riboflavin	0.119	mg
Niacin	0.869	mg
Pyridoxine (Vitamin B6)	0.126	mg
Folate (Total)	26.231	µg
Cobalamin (Vitamin B12)	0.000	µg
Pantothenic Acid	0.857	mg
Vitamin K	34.450	µg
Phosphorus	128.137	mg
Magnesium	53.077	mg
Zinc	0.418	mg
Copper	0.244	mg
Manganese	0.703	mg
Selenium	1.163	µg

Combine all ingredients, and mix until clumps have dissolved.

Heat a nonstick skillet or griddle pan over medium heat. Pour batter into the pan, forming 3-inch circles. When pancakes begin to bubble, flip and cook on the other side until lightly browned on both sides. Serve warm, topped with unsalted butter.

Serves 2.

Recipe Tidbit:

I have been able to find organic pumpkin in 15-ounce cartons. If you can find pumpkin in a carton, it may be a cleaner version than the canned variety. Alternatively, when pumpkins are in season, you can buy a pumpkin, bake or steam it, and scrape out the flesh. Fresh pumpkin is the tastiest option.

Recipe Tidbit:

Instead of a pan manufactured with a nonstick coating, I use a very well cured cast-iron pan.

Note that these gluten-free pancakes won't bubble as much as regular wheat-flour pancakes. If you wait until the pancakes produce as many bubbles as you are used to before flipping them, you may burn them. After flipping them, I sometimes flip them back to the first side for a minute or so to ensure that they have cooked all the way through.

SWEET POTATO HASH

INGREDIENTS

2 large sweet potatoes, cubed

1 small red onion, chopped

2 cloves garlic, minced

1 shallot, minced

3 tablespoons olive oil

1 red bell pepper, seeded and
chopped

1 tablespoon fresh rosemary,
minced

2 cups kale, stems removed, cut
into chiffonade

salt and pepper to taste

4 tablespoons fresh parsley,
minced

Macronutrients		
Kilocalories	137.484	kcal
Protein	2.226	g
Carbohydrate	5.706	g
Fat, Total	7.253	g
Alcohol	0.000	g
Cholesterol	0.000	mg
Saturated Fat	1.037	g
Monounsaturated Fat	4.951	g
Polyunsaturated Fat	0.869	g
Trans Fatty Acid	0.000	g
Dietary Fiber, Total	1.739	g
Sugar, Total	5.510	g
Percentage of Kcals		
Protein	9.2%	
Carbohydrate	23.5%	
Fat, total	67.3%	
Alcohol	0.0%	
Vitamins & Minerals		
Sodium	34.708	mg
Potassium	414.075	mg
Vitamin A (RE)	678.966	RE
Vitamin C	70.415	mg
Calcium	59.812	mg
Iron	1.104	mg
Vitamin D (ug)	0.000	µg
Vitamin E (mg)	0.159	mg
Thiamin	0.145	mg
Riboflavin	0.055	mg
Niacin	0.769	mg
Pyridoxine (Vitamin B6)	0.213	mg
Folate (Total)	58.564	µg
Cobalamin (Vitamin B12)	0.000	µg
Pantothenic Acid	0.441	mg
Vitamin K	204.091	µg
Phosphorus	63.600	mg
Magnesium	27.101	mg
Zinc	0.424	mg
Copper	0.434	mg
Manganese	0.425	mg
Selenium	1.044	µg

Preheat oven to 400°F. Add 1–2 inches of water to a baking pan, add cubed sweet potatoes, and bake for 25–35 minutes until tender.

In a large skillet, sauté onion, garlic, and shallot in olive oil for 2 minutes. Add red pepper and rosemary, and sauté another 3 minutes. Add sweet potatoes, kale, and salt and pepper, and sauté until mixture is combined and flavors begin to mingle, about 3–5 minutes. Top with fresh parsley and serve warm. If desired, prepare a poached or lightly fried egg and serve on top of the hash.

Serves 6.

Recipe Tidbit:

Always feel free to make substitutions as appropriate. You can use yams instead of sweet potatoes, but continue to stay away from white, yellow, purple, or red potatoes. Use fresh chives on top instead of parsley, or try a different herb instead of rosemary if you desire. Instead of the red pepper, you can try a green pepper—or any other variety you find appealing.

SQUASH PANCAKES

INGREDIENTS

2 cups butternut squash, steamed,
   cubed

4 eggs

½ cup hemp seeds, ground fine

¼ cup flaxseeds, ground fine

2 tablespoons coconut oil, melted

¼ teaspoon salt

½ teaspoon baking powder

Macronutrients		
Kilocalories	654.508	kcal
Protein	31.160	g
Carbohydrate	29.538	g
Fat, Total	48.183	g
Alcohol	0.000	g
Cholesterol	372.000	mg
Saturated Fat	17.186	g
Monounsaturated Fat	4.457	g
Polyunsaturated Fat	2.215	g
Trans Fatty Acid	0.038	g
Dietary Fiber, Total	11.602	g
Sugar, Total	3.450	g

Percentage of Kcals	
Protein	18.4%
Carbohydrate	17.5%
Fat, total	64.1%
Alcohol	0.0%

Vitamins & Minerals		
Sodium	566.852	mg
Potassium	1051.090	mg
Vitamin A (RE)	1650.216	RE
Vitamin C	29.400	mg
Calcium	244.287	mg
Iron	7.905	mg
Vitamin D (ug)	2.000	µg
Vitamin E (mg)	1.052	mg
Thiamin	0.180	mg
Riboflavin	0.485	mg
Niacin	1.755	mg
Pyridoxine (Vitamin B6)	0.386	mg
Folate (Total)	84.800	µg
Cobalamin (Vitamin B12)	0.890	µg
Pantothenic Acid	2.093	mg
Vitamin K	1.908	µg
Phosphorus	269.397	mg
Magnesium	331.918	mg
Zinc	1.501	mg
Copper	0.173	mg
Manganese	4.312	mg
Selenium	31.403	µg

Combine all ingredients and mix until clumps have dissolved.

Heat a nonstick skillet or griddle pan over medium heat. Pour batter into the pan, forming 3-inch circles. When pancakes begin to bubble, flip and cook on the other side until lightly browned on both sides. Serve warm, topped with unsalted butter and berries.

Serves 2.

Recipe Tidbit:

Instead of a pan manufactured with a nonstick coating, I use a very well cured cast-iron pan.

Note that these gluten-free pancakes won't bubble as much as regular wheat-flour pancakes. If you wait until the pancakes produce as many bubbles as you are used to before flipping them, you may burn them. After flipping them, I sometimes flip them back to the first side for a minute or so to ensure that they have cooked all the way through.

QUINOA GRANOLA

INGREDIENTS

½ cup sesame seeds

½ cup hemp seeds

½ cup flaxseeds

½ cup chia seeds

½ cup cooked quinoa (see recipe
   for cooked quinoa, page 85)

1 teaspoon cinnamon

½ teaspoon cardamom

2 large eggs or 3 small eggs, lightly
   beaten with a fork

1 teaspoon vanilla extract

Macronutrients		
Kilocalories	325.139	kcal
Protein	14.204	g
Carbohydrate	18.831	g
Fat, Total	22.712	g
Alcohol	0.241	g
Cholesterol	62.000	mg
Saturated Fat	2.816	g
Monounsaturated Fat	3.252	g
Polyunsaturated Fat	6.254	g
Trans Fatty Acid	0.025	g
Dietary Fiber, Total	11.617	g
Sugar, Total	0.329	g

Percentage of Kcals	
Protein	16.8%
Carbohydrate	22.3%
Fat, total	60.4%
Alcohol	0.5%

Vitamins & Minerals		
Sodium	32.774	mg
Potassium	304.440	mg
Vitamin A (RE)	27.781	RE
Vitamin C	0.262	mg
Calcium	253.181	mg
Iron	5.272	mg
Vitamin D (ug)	0.333	µg
Vitamin E (mg)	0.175	mg
Thiamin	0.201	mg
Riboflavin	0.147	mg
Niacin	1.805	mg
Pyridoxine (Vitamin B6)	0.235	mg
Folate (Total)	32.505	µg
Cobalamin (Vitamin B12)	0.148	µg
Pantothenic Acid	0.388	mg
Vitamin K	0.170	µg
Phosphorus	247.157	mg
Magnesium	190.005	mg
Zinc	1.944	mg
Copper	0.657	mg
Manganese	2.207	mg
Selenium	17.082	µg

Preheat oven to 350°F. Thoroughly mix together all dry ingredients. Add the eggs and vanilla, and combine until uniform. Spread on a baking sheet and bake until the mixture has browned, about 15–20 minutes. Every 5 minutes while baking, remove the mixture from the oven and stir. Remove from oven, allow to cool, and store in airtight container. Serve with unsweetened almond milk topped with berries of your choice.

Serves 6.

Recipe Tidbit:

You can try adding a small amount of stevia to the granola and mixing it thoroughly after baking. I tend not to like the taste of stevia; therefore you won't see it listed in many of my recipes. I prefer to add a natural sweetness by adding berries.

LEFTOVER VEGGIES WITH EGGS

You will notice that this recipe doesn't list nutritional information. That's because it can be made with so many variations. Part of my purpose in this book is to teach you how to improvise in the kitchen and how to avoid letting food go to waste. This recipe offers examples of foods that you can easily convert to a delicious egg scramble in the morning.

INGREDIENTS

2 cups leftover cooked veggies, chopped (e.g., broccoli, celery, peppers, zucchini, carrots)

1 tablespoon olive oil

6 eggs, lightly beaten

1 cup leafy greens (these could be kale, chard, collard greens, spinach)

salt and pepper to taste

Macronutrients		
Kilocalories	164.752	kcal
Protein	11.255	g
Carbohydrate	6.102	g
Fat, Total	10.915	g
Alcohol	0.000	g
Cholesterol	279.000	mg
Saturated Fat	2.875	g
Monounsaturated Fat	5.239	g
Polyunsaturated Fat	1.956	g
Trans Fatty Acid	0.029	g
Dietary Fiber, Total	2.050	g
Sugar, Total	2.805	g

Percentage of Kcals	
Protein	26.9%
Carbohydrate	14.6%
Fat, total	58.6%
Alcohol	0.0%

Vitamins & Minerals		
Sodium	139.230	mg
Potassium	403.577	mg
Vitamin A (RE)	336.755	RE
Vitamin C	50.417	mg
Calcium	89.763	mg
Iron	1.976	mg
Vitamin D (ug)	1.500	µg
Vitamin E (mg)	0.789	mg
Thiamin	0.086	mg
Riboflavin	0.414	mg
Niacin	0.635	mg
Pyridoxine (Vitamin B6)	0.292	mg
Folate (Total)	97.235	µg
Cobalamin (Vitamin B12)	0.668	µg
Biotin	0.098	µg
Pantothenic Acid	1.444	mg
Vitamin K	157.839	µg
Phosphorus	195.822	mg
Magnesium	30.617	mg
Zinc	1.295	mg
Copper	0.350	mg
Manganese	0.261	mg
Selenium	23.786	µg
Chromium	0.007	mg

Heat olive oil in a large skillet, and lightly sauté vegetables over medium heat. Add eggs, greens, salt, and pepper, and sauté until eggs are cooked to desired doneness.

Serves 4.

Recipe Tidbit:

Add anything you want to this scramble. If you can tolerate dairy, adding cheese will make it even more delicious. Consider adding feta, cheddar, Swiss, or another variety.

SAVORY QUINOA BREAKFAST BOWL

INGREDIENTS

1 cup cooked quinoa, warmed
  (see recipe for cooked quinoa on
  page 85)

4 eggs

1 tablespoon coconut oil, divided

1 cup kale, stems removed,
  chopped

4 tablespoons chopped cilantro

1 avocado, cubed

salt and pepper to taste

Macronutrients		
Kilocalories	220.558	kcal
Protein	9.708	g
Carbohydrate	14.601	g
Fat, Total	14.354	g
Alcohol	0.000	g
Cholesterol	186.000	mg
Saturated Fat	5.337	g
Monounsaturated Fat	5.554	g
Polyunsaturated Fat	2.179	g
Trans Fatty Acid	0.019	g
Dietary Fiber, Total	4.199	g
Sugar, Total	1.066	g

Percentage of Kcals	
Protein	17.2%
Carbohydrate	25.8%
Fat, total	57.1%
Alcohol	0.0%

Vitamins & Minerals		
Sodium	83.276	mg
Potassium	400.234	mg
Vitamin A (RE)	253.484	RE
Vitamin C	23.041	mg
Calcium	65.332	mg
Iron	2.016	mg
Vitamin D (ug)	1.000	µg
Vitamin E (mg)	0.526	mg
Thiamin	0.113	mg
Riboflavin	0.349	mg
Niacin	1.035	mg
Pyridoxine (Vitamin B6)	0.283	mg
Folate (Total)	96.287	µg
Cobalamin (Vitamin B12)	0.445	µg
Pantothenic Acid	1.271	mg
Vitamin K	125.239	µg
Phosphorus	202.757	mg
Magnesium	53.164	mg
Zinc	1.470	mg
Copper	0.433	mg
Manganese	0.466	mg
Selenium	16.929	µg

Lightly steam kale until it is bright green. In a small skillet, warm ¼ of the coconut oil to medium heat, and crack an egg into the pan. Cook until the egg white turns white but the yolk is still soft. Flip and cook for another minute or until you reach desired yolk hardness. Repeat with the 3 remaining eggs.

Divide the warm quinoa among 4 individual serving bowls, top each with ¼ of the kale, then layer a cooked egg over the top of each. Top each serving with avocado and cilantro, and season as desired with salt and pepper.

Serves 4.

QUINOA BREAKFAST BOWL

INGREDIENTS

1 cup cooked quinoa (see recipe
   for cooked quinoa on page 85)

1 cup unsweetened almond milk

½ cup pecans

1 teaspoon cinnamon

½ teaspoon nutmeg

½ teaspoon carob powder

1 cup raspberries

1 avocado, cubed

salt to taste

In a saucepan, combine all ingredients except berries and avocado; gently heat until warm. Transfer to 4 individual serving bowls, and top each with avocado and berries. Serve warm.

Macronutrients		
Kilocalories	247.407	kcal
Protein	6.610	g
Carbohydrate	20.385	g
Fat, Total	17.278	g
Alcohol	0.000	g
Cholesterol	0.000	mg
Saturated Fat	1.864	g
Monounsaturated Fat	9.359	g
Polyunsaturated Fat	4.793	g
Trans Fatty Acid	0.000	g
Dietary Fiber, Total	8.343	g
Sugar, Total	2.804	g
Percentage of Kcals		
Protein	10.0%	
Carbohydrate	30.9%	
Fat, total	59.0%	
Alcohol	0.0%	
Vitamins & Minerals		
Sodium	13.913	mg
Potassium	431.933	mg
Vitamin A (RE)	7.119	RE
Vitamin C	11.178	mg
Calcium	46.773	mg
Iron	1.970	mg
Vitamin D (ug)	0.000	µg
Thiamin	0.176	mg
Riboflavin	0.130	mg
Niacin	1.189	mg
Pyridoxine (Vitamin B6)	0.201	mg
Folate (Total)	58.945	µg
Cobalamin (Vitamin B12)	0.000	µg
Biotin	0.585	µg
Pantothenic Acid	0.710	mg
Vitamin K	10.073	µg
Phosphorus	136.170	mg
Magnesium	63.535	mg
Zinc	1.497	mg
Copper	0.343	mg
Manganese	1.269	mg
Selenium	2.044	µg

Serves 4.

Recipe Tidbit:

This dish can easily be made ahead of time and enjoyed warm or cold. If you're eating it cold and it seems too thick, add a little more milk.

PEACH COCONUT PORRIDGE

INGREDIENTS

1 cup brown rice, rinsed twice

1 tablespoon apple cider vinegar

6 cups filtered water

2 cups chopped fresh peaches

½ cup unsweetened shredded coconut

1 teaspoon cinnamon

½ teaspoon nutmeg

¼ teaspoon salt

1 tablespoon unsweetened sunflower butter (optional)

Combine rice, apple cider vinegar, and water in slow cooker, and soak during the day for about 12 hours. Add remaining ingredients; cook on low overnight for 12 hours. Your porridge will be ready in the morning.

Macronutrients		
Kilocalories	169.868	kcal
Protein	3.275	g
Carbohydrate	30.469	g
Fat, Total	4.433	g
Alcohol	0.000	g
Cholesterol	0.000	mg
Saturated Fat	3.239	g
Monounsaturated Fat	0.367	g
Polyunsaturated Fat	0.367	g
Trans Fatty Acid	0.000	g
Dietary Fiber, Total	2.758	g
Sugar, Total	4.926	g
Percentage of Kcals		
Protein	7.5%	
Carbohydrate	69.7%	
Fat, total	22.8%	
Alcohol	0.0%	
Vitamins & Minerals		
Sodium	108.022	mg
Potassium	172.788	mg
Vitamin A (RE)	16.866	RE
Vitamin C	3.408	mg
Calcium	21.694	mg
Iron	0.745	mg
Vitamin D (ug)	0.000	µg
Thiamin	0.137	mg
Riboflavin	0.045	mg
Niacin	1.991	mg
Pyridoxine (Vitamin B6)	0.171	mg
Folate (Total)	8.382	µg
Cobalamin (Vitamin B12)	0.000	µg
Biotin	1.027	µg
Pantothenic Acid	0.540	mg
Vitamin K	2.040	µg
Phosphorus	113.776	mg
Magnesium	51.774	mg
Zinc	0.722	mg
Copper	0.145	mg
Manganese	1.264	mg
Selenium	7.284	µg
Chromium	0.001	mg

Serves: 6

Recipe tidbit:

This recipe requires very little prep time and is extremely easy if planned out correctly. Start the process on one morning for warm porridge the next. For a higher-protein version, substitute 2 cups of quinoa for the rice, using the same amount of water. (Quinoa absorbs less water than brown rice.) I suggest avoiding grains as much as you can while on this diet, so let this simple dish be a treat for you. The long, slow soaking and cooking make the grain very digestible.

SCOTCH EGGS

INGREDIENTS

4 soft-boiled eggs

1 pound bulk chicken sausage or turkey sausage (look at ingredients to ensure there is no sugar)

1 tablespoon sunflower seeds, ground

pinch salt and pepper

1 egg, lightly beaten

¼ cup grated Parmesan

3 tablespoons hemp seeds, ground

3 tablespoons coconut oil

1 head butter lettuce

Macronutrients		
Kilocalories	453.133	kcal
Protein	35.443	g
Carbohydrate	3.404	g
Fat, Total	33.423	g
Alcohol	0.000	g
Cholesterol	333.998	mg
Saturated Fat	15.197	g
Monounsaturated Fat	3.654	g
Polyunsaturated Fat	2.016	g
Trans Fatty Acid	0.024	g
Dietary Fiber, Total	1.167	g
Sugar, Total	0.677	g
Percentage of Kcals		
Protein	31.1%	
Carbohydrate	3.0%	
Fat, total	65.9%	
Alcohol	0.0%	
Vitamins & Minerals		
Sodium	796.779	mg
Potassium	285.498	mg
Vitamin A (RE)	242.968	RE
Vitamin C	1.539	mg
Calcium	93.668	mg
Iron	3.722	mg
Vitamin D (ug)	1.275	µg
Vitamin E (mg)	0.837	mg
Thiamin	0.083	mg
Riboflavin	0.337	mg
Niacin	0.384	mg
Pyridoxine (Vitamin B6)	0.174	mg
Folate (Total)	64.530	µg
Cobalamin (Vitamin B12)	0.626	µg
Biotin	1.373	µg
Pantothenic Acid	1.067	mg
Vitamin K	42.011	µg
Phosphorus	183.398	mg
Magnesium	72.810	mg
Zinc	1.210	mg
Copper	0.094	mg
Manganese	0.888	mg
Selenium	22.345	µg
Chromium	0.011	mg
Molybdenum	0.969	µg

To soft-boil eggs: Place the egg(s) in a large saucepan, and add room-temperature water, covering to at least 1–2 inches above the top of the egg(s). Bring the water to boil over medium to high heat. Once the water is boiling, cover with a lid and remove from heat. Allow the eggs to sit for 1–2 minutes. Transfer them to a large colander, and rinse with cold water to stop further cooking. Peel and serve. Refrigerate them in their shells if you plan to use them later.

Preheat oven to 400ºF. In a medium bowl, mix together the sausage with ground sunflower seeds, salt, and pepper. Divide the sausage mixture into 4 equal portions. Mold each portion around 1 soft-boiled egg. Combine the Parmesan and ground hemp seeds. Dip each sausage-wrapped egg in the beaten egg, and then roll it through the Parmesan–hemp mixture, coating the egg as evenly as possible.

In a skillet over medium heat, heat the coconut oil. Cook each of the eggs, turning often enough to brown all sides. Transfer eggs to a baking pan, place in oven, and bake until sausage is cooked, about 15–25 minutes. Remove from the oven and allow to cool slightly. Divide leaves of butter lettuce evenly among 4 plates, arranging so that the leaves form a bowl shape. Place 1 scotch egg onto each lettuce bowl, and serve immediately.

Serves 4.

Recipe Tidbit:

Scotch eggs are typically fried; this recipe offers a healthier but still delicious alternative. For an even healthier version, cover the scotch eggs while baking them to retain moisture. As I explained in *The Freedom Diet,* cooking meats using a moist-heat method produces fewer damaging oxidative compounds.

CHIA FLAX PUDDING

INGREDIENTS

½ cup chia seeds

2 tablespoons flaxseeds

1 cup unsweetened almond milk

1 cup full-fat coconut milk

1 teaspoon vanilla extract

½ teaspoon carob

½ teaspoon cardamom

very small pinch salt

Fresh raspberries, blueberries, and blackberries

Macronutrients		
Kilocalories	288.741	kcal
Protein	7.971	g
Carbohydrate	15.367	g
Fat, Total	23.429	g
Alcohol	0.361	g
Cholesterol	0.000	mg
Saturated Fat	13.644	g
Monounsaturated Fat	1.323	g
Polyunsaturated Fat	5.516	g
Trans Fatty Acid	0.028	g
Dietary Fiber, Total	10.874	g
Sugar, Total	2.518	g
Percentage of Kcals		
Protein	10.4%	
Carbohydrate	20.0%	
Fat, total	68.7%	
Alcohol	0.8%	
Vitamins & Minerals		
Sodium	21.598	mg
Potassium	320.673	mg
Vitamin A (RE)	0.720	RE
Vitamin C	2.051	mg
Calcium	161.253	mg
Iron	3.207	mg
Vitamin D (ug)	0.000	µg
Thiamin	0.140	mg
Riboflavin	0.037	mg
Niacin	2.234	mg
Pyridoxine (Vitamin B6)	0.160	mg
Folate (Total)	19.478	µg
Cobalamin (Vitamin B12)	0.000	µg
Pantothenic Acid	0.298	mg
Vitamin K	0.060	µg
Phosphorus	232.708	mg
Magnesium	90.026	mg
Zinc	1.340	mg
Copper	0.348	mg
Manganese	1.164	mg
Selenium	14.825	µg

Whisk together all ingredients except the berries for at least 5 minutes, and pour into a large serving bowl or 4 individual serving glasses. Cover and store in the refrigerator until set, about ½ hour. Serve chilled, topped with berries.

Serves 4.

Recipe Tidbit:

This dish can easily be made the night before for a quick bite to eat in the morning.

Chapter 2

SNACKS, SIDES, APPETIZERS, AND CONDIMENTS

DEVILLED EGGS

INGREDIENTS

12 hard-boiled eggs

½ cup mayonnaise

1 tablespoon mustard

salt and pepper to taste

paprika and chopped fresh
dill for garnish

To hard-boil eggs: Place the egg(s) in a large saucepan, and add room-temperature water, covering to at least 1–2 inches above the top of the egg(s). Bring the water to boil over medium to high heat. Once the water is boiling, cover with a lid and remove from heat. Allow time for the eggs to continue cooking, about 10 minutes. After the eggs are cooked, if you want to eat them immediately, place them in a colander and rinse with cold water. Peel and serve. Otherwise, transfer the eggs to the refrigerator for future use.

Crack the eggshell, and roll the egg gently back and forth on the countertop. Carefully peel the eggs, rinse with cold water, and gently pat dry with paper towels. Slice each egg in half lengthwise; scoop the yolks into a medium bowl, and place the whites on a serving platter. Mash the yolks into a fine crumble using a fork. Add mayonnaise, mustard, salt, and pepper, and mix well. Evenly disperse heaping

Macronutrients		
Kilocalories	281.620	kcal
Protein	12.850	g
Carbohydrate	1.371	g
Fat, Total	24.466	g
Alcohol	0.000	g
Cholesterol	380.728	mg
Saturated Fat	5.426	g
Monounsaturated Fat	7.231	g
Polyunsaturated Fat	9.656	g
Trans Fatty Acid	0.035	g
Dietary Fiber, Total	0.100	g
Sugar, Total	1.248	g

Percentage of Kcals	
Protein	18.6%
Carbohydrate	2.0%
Fat, total	79.5%
Alcohol	0.0%

Vitamins & Minerals		
Sodium	268.440	mg
Potassium	133.480	mg
Vitamin A (RE)	158.586	RE
Vitamin C	0.008	mg
Calcium	53.047	mg
Iron	1.269	mg
Vitamin D (ug)	2.237	µg
Thiamin	0.072	mg
Riboflavin	0.518	mg
Niacin	0.078	mg
Pyridoxine (Vitamin B6)	0.124	mg
Folate (Total)	45.095	µg
Cobalamin (Vitamin B12)	1.132	µg
Biotin	22.173	µg
Pantothenic Acid	1.436	mg
Vitamin K	30.327	µg
Phosphorus	178.564	mg
Magnesium	11.384	mg
Zinc	1.094	mg
Copper	0.018	mg
Manganese	0.038	mg
Selenium	32.061	µg
Chromium	0.006	mg

teaspoons of the yolk mixture into the egg whites. Sprinkle with paprika and dill and serve.

Serves 6.

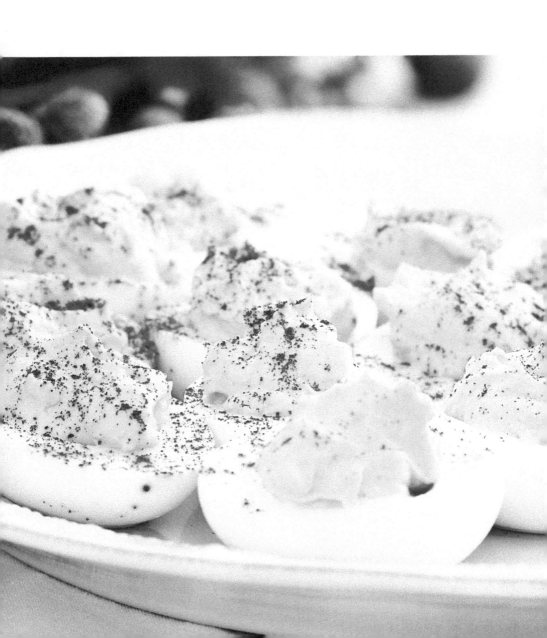

ROASTED BEANS

INGREDIENTS

1 pound green beans, washed and trimmed

1 15-ounce can navy or white beans, drained

2 tablespoons olive oil

1 teaspoon garlic powder

1 teaspoon onion powder

½ teaspoon cumin powder

½ teaspoon salt

½ teaspoon pepper

Macronutrients		
Kilocalories	221.071	kcal
Protein	10.328	g
Carbohydrate	30.837	g
Fat, Total	7.526	g
Alcohol	0.000	g
Cholesterol	0.000	mg
Saturated Fat	1.114	g
Monounsaturated Fat	4.980	g
Polyunsaturated Fat	1.042	g
Trans Fatty Acid	0.000	g
Dietary Fiber, Total	8.793	g
Sugar, Total	4.048	g
Percentage of Kcals		
Protein	17.8%	
Carbohydrate	53.1%	
Fat, total	29.1%	
Alcohol	0.0%	
Vitamins & Minerals		
Sodium	775.011	mg
Potassium	544.106	mg
Vitamin A (RE)	70.769	RE
Vitamin C	11.251	mg
Calcium	96.305	mg
Iron	3.202	mg
Vitamin D (ug)	0.000	µg
Thiamin	0.230	mg
Riboflavin	0.166	mg
Niacin	1.235	mg
Pyridoxine (Vitamin B6)	0.262	mg
Folate (Total)	90.946	µg
Cobalamin (Vitamin B12)	0.000	µg
Pantothenic Acid	0.451	mg
Vitamin K	23.930	µg
Phosphorus	186.242	mg
Magnesium	78.487	mg
Zinc	1.123	mg
Copper	0.306	mg
Manganese	0.692	mg
Selenium	7.102	µg
Chromium	0.001	mg

Preheat oven to 400ºF. In a large bowl, whisk together olive oil and spices until thoroughly mixed. Add green beans, tossing to coat with the oil mixture. Transfer beans to a roasting pan, place in oven, and roast until beans are still bright green but tender, about 10–15 minutes. Remove from oven, combine with navy or white beans, and return to oven. Roast for another 5 minutes. Serve warm.

Serves 4.

JICAMA WITH LIME

INGREDIENTS

1 large jicama
2 teaspoons fresh lime juice
pinch salt

Peel jicama and cut into 1-inch chunks. Toss with lime, sprinkle with a small amount of salt, and serve chilled.

Serves 2.

Macronutrients		
Kilocalories	126.493	kcal
Protein	2.394	g
Carbohydrate	29.494	g
Fat, Total	0.300	g
Alcohol	0.000	g
Cholesterol	0.000	mg
Saturated Fat	0.070	g
Monounsaturated Fat	0.017	g
Polyunsaturated Fat	0.143	g
Trans Fatty Acid		g
Dietary Fiber, Total	16.166	g
Sugar, Total	6.018	g

Percentage of Kcals	
Protein	7.4%
Carbohydrate	90.6%
Fat, total	2.1%
Alcohol	0.0%

Vitamins & Minerals		
Sodium	27.817	mg
Potassium	500.259	mg
Vitamin A (RE)	7.176	RE
Vitamin C	68.099	mg
Calcium	40.268	mg
Iron	1.982	mg
Vitamin D (ug)	0.000	µg
Thiamin	0.067	mg
Riboflavin	0.096	mg
Niacin	0.666	mg
Pyridoxine (Vitamin B6)	0.140	mg
Folate (Total)	40.053	µg
Cobalamin (Vitamin B12)	0.000	µg
Pantothenic Acid	0.451	mg
Vitamin K	1.019	µg
Phosphorus	60.029	mg
Magnesium	39.951	mg
Zinc	0.531	mg
Copper	0.160	mg
Manganese	0.199	mg
Selenium	2.312	µg

CELERY AND SUNBUTTER

INGREDIENTS

4 large celery stalks, cut into 2-inch
  long sticks

3 cups raw sunflower seeds

¾ teaspoon salt

1 tablespoon olive oil

Macronutrients		
Kilocalories	166.739	kcal
Protein	5.680	g
Carbohydrate	5.697	g
Fat, Total	14.755	g
Alcohol	0.000	g
Cholesterol	0.000	mg
Saturated Fat	1.324	g
Monounsaturated Fat	5.621	g
Polyunsaturated Fat	6.344	g
Trans Fatty Acid		g
Dietary Fiber, Total	2.482	g
Sugar, Total	0.841	g
Percentage of Kcals		
Protein	12.7%	
Carbohydrate	12.8%	
Fat, total	74.5%	
Alcohol	0.0%	
Vitamins & Minerals		
Sodium	119.454	mg
Potassium	200.181	mg
Vitamin A (RE)	5.840	RE
Vitamin C	0.688	mg
Calcium	25.136	mg
Iron	1.443	mg
Vitamin D (ug)	0.000	µg
Thiamin	0.402	mg
Riboflavin	0.102	mg
Niacin	2.282	mg
Pyridoxine (Vitamin B6)	0.371	mg
Folate (Total)	64.890	µg
Cobalamin (Vitamin B12)	0.000	µg
Biotin	0.010	µg
Pantothenic Acid	0.330	mg
Vitamin K	3.438	µg
Phosphorus	180.600	mg
Magnesium	88.853	mg
Zinc	1.363	mg
Copper	0.490	mg
Manganese	0.537	mg
Selenium	14.350	µg
Chromium	0.001	mg
Molybdenum	0.167	µg

To prepare the sunbutter, place seeds in a large skillet, and cook over medium heat, stirring constantly, until lightly toasted, about 5 minutes. Process seeds in a food processor or blender until mixture appears smooth and oily, about 10 minutes. Add salt, and continue processing until mixture is the consistency of smooth peanut butter, about 5 minutes. With food processor running, slowly drizzle in olive oil, processing until very smooth. Spread the sunbutter evenly onto the celery sticks, and enjoy immediately. Alternatively, spoon the sunbutter into a jar, and store for use later.

Warning: the long processing time can leave the mixture hot enough to burn the skin. Use caution when handling.

Serves 16.

Recipe Tidbit:

You can find sunflower-seed butter online or in some grocery stores, but make sure you purchase a version that does not have added sugar.

CUCUMBER CREAM-CHEESE SANDWICHES

INGREDIENTS

2 large cucumbers, sliced

½ cup cream cheese

fresh dill, chopped

Arrange half the cucumber slices on a serving dish, and top each slice with a small amount of cream cheese and fresh dill to taste. Top with another slice of cucumber, completing the cucumber sandwich.

Serves 2.

Recipe Tidbit:

I included this very simple recipe to help you start thinking about how to improvise with ingredients you have on hand to make snacks that are simple and healthy and that don't contain sugar or bread. Using this same idea, substitute other ingredients that are in your pantry and refrigerator. Sometimes I put out a large platter of snacks with toothpicks, and my daughters make tall "sandwiches" from the supplied ingredients. Consider using sliced red or green bell pepper, cherry tomatoes, slices of cheese, slices of baked chicken. . . . You get the idea.

Macronutrients

Kilocalories	243.530	kcal
Protein	5.398	g
Carbohydrate	13.290	g
Fat, Total	20.191	g
Alcohol	0.000	g
Cholesterol	63.800	mg
Saturated Fat	11.301	g
Monounsaturated Fat	5.015	g
Polyunsaturated Fat	0.930	g
Trans Fatty Acid		g
Dietary Fiber, Total	1.506	g
Sugar, Total	6.889	g

Percentage of Kcals

Protein	8.4%
Carbohydrate	20.7%
Fat, total	70.9%
Alcohol	0.0%

Vitamins & Minerals

Sodium	217.749	mg
Potassium	522.854	mg
Vitamin A (RE)	252.097	RE
Vitamin C	8.468	mg
Calcium	105.097	mg
Iron	1.066	mg
Vitamin D (ug)	0.348	µg
Thiamin	0.093	mg
Riboflavin	0.172	mg
Niacin	0.380	mg
Pyridoxine (Vitamin B6)	0.141	mg
Folate (Total)	27.520	µg
Cobalamin (Vitamin B12)	0.145	µg
Biotin	0.808	µg
Pantothenic Acid	1.110	mg
Vitamin K	51.046	µg
Phosphorus	133.751	mg
Magnesium	44.376	mg
Zinc	0.898	mg
Copper	0.134	mg
Manganese	0.245	mg
Selenium	2.295	µg
Molybdenum	2.636	µg

SPICY SEED CRACKERS

INGREDIENTS

½ cup sesame seeds

¼ cup hemp seeds

¼ cup sunflower seeds

¼ cup pumpkin seeds

1 cup water

1 egg, lightly beaten with a fork

3 cloves garlic, minced fine

1 shallot, minced fine

½ teaspoon black pepper

½ teaspoon thyme

¼ teaspoon salt

¼ teaspoon cayenne pepper

¼ teaspoon rosemary

Macronutrients		
Kilocalories	284.689	kcal
Protein	12.805	g
Carbohydrate	9.790	g
Fat, Total	23.457	g
Alcohol	0.000	g
Cholesterol	46.500	mg
Saturated Fat	3.211	g
Monounsaturated Fat	6.911	g
Polyunsaturated Fat	8.072	g
Trans Fatty Acid	0.010	g
Dietary Fiber, Total	4.436	g
Sugar, Total	0.692	g

Percentage of Kcals	
Protein	17.0%
Carbohydrate	13.0%
Fat, total	70.0%
Alcohol	0.0%

Vitamins & Minerals		
Sodium	169.166	mg
Potassium	360.206	mg
Vitamin A (RE)	26.692	RE
Vitamin C	1.411	mg
Calcium	205.949	mg
Iron	5.493	mg
Vitamin D (ug)	0.250	µg
Vitamin E (mg)	0.132	mg
Thiamin	0.312	mg
Riboflavin	0.152	mg
Niacin	2.045	mg
Pyridoxine (Vitamin B6)	0.339	mg
Folate (Total)	50.559	µg
Cobalamin (Vitamin B12)	0.111	µg
Pantothenic Acid	0.391	mg
Vitamin K	4.246	µg
Phosphorus	309.807	mg
Magnesium	215.844	mg
Zinc	2.735	mg
Copper	1.042	mg
Manganese	2.110	mg
Selenium	15.994	µg
Chromium	0.003	mg

Preheat oven to 350ºF. Combine all ingredients in a large bowl. Line a 9 x 13–inch baking sheet with parchment paper so that the paper overlaps all edges of the pan (the mixture will have a somewhat liquid consistency). Pour entire mixture onto the parchment paper and spread evenly. Bake for 30 minutes. Remove the pan from the oven, and carefully cut the baked mixture into 1- to 2-inch squares. Flip each cracker over, and bake for another 20 minutes until crackers are crispy on the edges. Remove from oven, and use a spatula to move the crackers onto a baking cloth to dry. When completely cool, transfer to an airtight container to store.

Serves 4.

Recipe Tidbit:

Although this recipe makes crackers that are only mildly spicy, if you want even less spice, simply eliminate the cayenne pepper and slightly reduce the amount of black pepper and garlic used.

On this diet, you may find yourself missing carbohydrate snacks such as chips and crackers. These little crackers help satisfy that craving for crunchy carbs, and their rich seed content makes them better at helping to curb your appetite. In addition, seeds are packed with protein, which can help to regulate blood sugar. Try dipping these crackers in hummus or eating them with sliced cucumber or yellow beets.

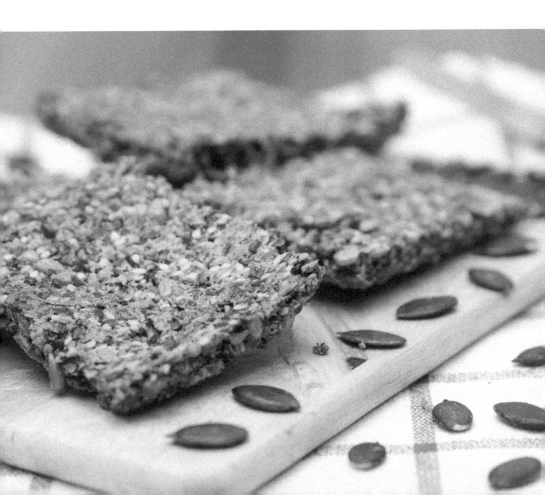

KALE CHIPS

INGREDIENTS

1 bunch kale, stems removed,
   chopped into 1- to 2-inch pieces

1 tablespoon olive oil

½ teaspoon salt

Preheat oven to 300ºF. Combine kale with olive oil and salt in a large mixing bowl, and stir until thoroughly combined. Arrange the kale on 2 or 3 parchment paper–lined baking pans. Make sure the kale is spread evenly to make a single layer rather than bunched up. Bake for 10 minutes, remove the pans from the oven, stir the kale, and place back in the oven. Bake for another 10 minutes or so, just until the kale starts to brown on its edges. Transfer to a large bowl, and set out for snacking.

Serves 6.

Macronutrients		
Kilocalories	36.305	kcal
Protein	1.434	g
Carbohydrate	2.931	g
Fat, Total	2.562	g
Alcohol	0.000	g
Cholesterol	0.000	mg
Saturated Fat	0.341	g
Monounsaturated Fat	1.659	g
Polyunsaturated Fat	0.350	g
Trans Fatty Acid		g
Dietary Fiber, Total	1.206	g
Sugar, Total	0.757	g

Percentage of Kcals	
Protein	14.2%
Carbohydrate	28.9%
Fat, total	56.9%
Alcohol	0.0%

Vitamins & Minerals		
Sodium	206.565	mg
Potassium	164.548	mg
Vitamin A (RE)	334.665	RE
Vitamin C	40.200	mg
Calcium	50.393	mg
Iron	0.507	mg
Vitamin D (ug)	0.000	µg
Thiamin	0.037	mg
Riboflavin	0.044	mg
Niacin	0.335	mg
Pyridoxine (Vitamin B6)	0.091	mg
Folate (Total)	47.235	µg
Cobalamin (Vitamin B12)	0.000	µg
Pantothenic Acid	0.030	mg
Vitamin K	237.463	µg
Phosphorus	30.820	mg
Magnesium	15.750	mg
Zinc	0.188	mg
Copper	0.502	mg
Manganese	0.221	mg
Selenium	0.302	µg

Recipe Tidbit:

It is important to avoid overcooking the kale. Remember that even after you remove the kale from the oven, if left on the pans, it will continue to cook. I always err on the side of undercooking it and then allow it to rest on the pans for a little bit until it has reached the desired crispness.

You can keep this recipe basic and simple, or you can get very creative by adding additional ingredients such as nutritional yeast, onion or garlic powders, cayenne, mustard powder, cumin, or other seasonings.

MY FAVORITE RELISH PLATE WITH HUMMUS

INGREDIENTS

2 green bell peppers, one sliced
and one whole

1 yellow bell pepper, sliced

1 red bell pepper, sliced

1 bunch radishes, cleaned and sliced

1 cup cubed jicama

1 cucumber, cut into long, thin
sticks

1 carrot, cut into long, thin sticks

1 10-ounce jar whole, pitted
kalamata olives (no sugar added)

1 pint cherry tomatoes

1 can pitted black olives (no sugar
added)

1 cup feta cheese, cut into chunks
(optional)

Macronutrients		
Kilocalories	426.767	kcal
Protein	8.022	g
Carbohydrate	35.893	g
Fat, Total	29.179	g
Alcohol	0.000	g
Cholesterol	0.000	mg
Saturated Fat	2.342	g
Monounsaturated Fat	11.169	g
Polyunsaturated Fat	2.354	g
Trans Fatty Acid	0.000	g
Dietary Fiber, Total	8.254	g
Sugar, Total	6.308	g
Percentage of Kcals		
Protein	7.3%	
Carbohydrate	32.8%	
Fat, total	59.9%	
Alcohol	0.0%	
Vitamins & Minerals		
Sodium	1426.893	mg
Potassium	692.586	mg
Vitamin A (RE)	268.330	RE
Vitamin C	133.958	mg
Calcium	89.814	mg
Iron	3.126	mg
Vitamin D (ug)	0.000	µg
Thiamin	0.233	mg
Riboflavin	0.121	mg
Niacin	1.712	mg
Pyridoxine (Vitamin B6)	0.386	mg
Folate (Total)	87.265	µg
Cobalamin (Vitamin B12)	0.000	µg
Biotin	0.305	µg
Pantothenic Acid	0.493	mg
Vitamin K	27.699	µg
Phosphorus	172.290	mg
Magnesium	64.578	mg
Zinc	1.153	mg
Copper	0.386	mg
Manganese	0.466	mg
Selenium	5.787	µg
Chromium	0.008	mg
Molybdenum	0.878	µg

Simple White-Bean Hummus:

1 15-ounce can navy beans, drained, or 1½ cups cooked navy beans

1 tablespoon tahini

2 garlic cloves

¼ cup fresh lemon juice

⅓ cup olive oil

½ teaspoon salt

To prepare the hummus, in a food processor or high-powered blender blend together the tahini, garlic, lemon juice, and olive oil until smooth. Add salt and navy beans, and pulse minimally, leaving the hummus chunky. Refrigerate until needed to allow flavors to combine.

Cut the very top off of the whole green pepper, and remove the pith and the seeds. Fill the pepper with the hummus, and place in the center of a serving platter. Arrange the remaining ingredients around the hummus-filled pepper to create a beautiful relish tray.

Serves 6.

Recipe Tidbit:

Experiment with using as many different vegetables as you wish, for example, celery, broccoli, cauliflower, white mushrooms, and green onions.

ROASTED SQUASH RINGS

INGREDIENTS

3 delicata squash
¼ cup olive oil
salt and pepper to taste

Preheat oven to 400ºF. Wash squash well. Cut each squash in half, across its width. Cut off ends, and scoop out and discard seeds. Cut squash into ½-inch to ¾-inch thick rings. Toss with olive oil. Arrange squash on foil or parchment paper-lined baking sheet, and sprinkle lightly with salt and pepper.

Roast for 20–30 minutes until tender and lightly browned, turning halfway through cooking time.

Serves 6.

Macronutrients		
Kilocalories	86.653	kcal
Protein	0.377	g
Carbohydrate	1.449	g
Fat, Total	9.101	g
Alcohol	0.000	g
Cholesterol	0.000	mg
Saturated Fat	1.277	g
Monounsaturated Fat	6.571	g
Polyunsaturated Fat	0.978	g
Trans Fatty Acid	0.000	g
Dietary Fiber, Total	0.373	g
Sugar, Total	1.075	g

Percentage of Kcals	
Protein	1.7%
Carbohydrate	6.5%
Fat, total	91.8%
Alcohol	0.0%

Vitamins & Minerals		
Sodium	0.927	mg
Potassium	82.970	mg
Vitamin A (RE)	5.600	RE
Vitamin C	7.205	mg
Calcium	7.930	mg
Iron	0.215	mg
Vitamin D (ug)	0.000	µg
Thiamin	0.019	mg
Riboflavin	0.015	mg
Niacin	0.167	mg
Pyridoxine (Vitamin B6)	0.039	mg
Folate (Total)	7.093	µg
Cobalamin (Vitamin B12)	0.000	µg
Pantothenic Acid	0.060	mg
Vitamin K	6.613	µg
Phosphorus	11.947	mg
Magnesium	7.467	mg
Zinc	0.108	mg
Copper	0.034	mg
Manganese	0.064	mg
Selenium	0.075	µg

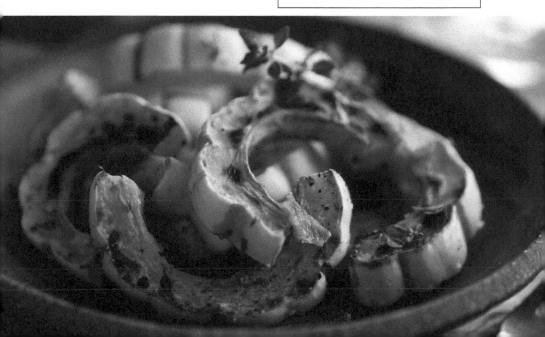

Recipe Tidbit:

Other types of winter squash can be used in this recipe as long as the skins are edible, for example, acorn or butternut. You can do some research online to see which varieties of squash fit this category. If you can't cut the squash into rings, I suggest cutting them into 1- to 2-inch cubes, seeds and pulp removed before roasting. Sprinkling the squash with rosemary prior to roasting adds delicious flavor.

Preliminary studies have shown winter squash to have anti-inflammatory benefits. Winter squash contains some fat, including the anti-inflammatory omega-3s, but it is not considered a high-fat food. One cup of baked winter squash provides approximately 340 milligrams of omega-3 fats in the form of alpha-linolenic acid (ALA). Squash also fit into the yellow-orange category of plant foods that are helpful at preventing heart disease. Finally, consuming winter squash is a good way to curb your sweet tooth. They can be a delicious sweet treat.

ROASTED VEGETABLES

INGREDIENTS

2 zucchini

2 yellow squash

1 red bell pepper

1 green bell pepper

1 red onion

2 large carrots

¼ cup olive oil

salt and pepper to taste

Preheat oven to 450°F. Cut vegetables into 1- to 2-inch pieces. Toss in large bowl with olive oil until coated. Arrange vegetables in single layer on two foil or parchment paper-lined sheet pans, and sprinkle lightly with salt and pepper. Roast for 30–45 minutes, stirring every 10 minutes, until vegetables are crisp-tender and starting to brown.

Serves 8.

Macronutrients		
Kilocalories	98.446	kcal
Trans Fatty Acid		g
Sugar, Total		g
Protein	1.665	g
Carbohydrate	8.239	g
Fat, Total	7.105	g
Alcohol	0.000	g
Cholesterol	0.000	mg
Saturated Fat	1.011	g
Monounsaturated Fat	4.941	g
Polyunsaturated Fat	0.824	g
Trans Fatty Acid	0.000	g
Dietary Fiber, Total	2.119	g
Sugar, Total	4.319	g
Percentage of Kcals		
Protein	6.4%	
Carbohydrate	31.8%	
Fat, total	61.7%	
Alcohol	0.0%	
Vitamins & Minerals		
Sodium	18.284	mg
Potassium	361.040	mg
Vitamin A (RE)	334.285	RE
Vitamin C	52.959	mg
Calcium	27.856	mg
Iron	0.720	mg
Vitamin D (ug)	0.000	µg
Thiamin	0.077	mg
Riboflavin	0.123	mg
Niacin	0.825	mg
Pyridoxine (Vitamin B6)	0.269	mg
Folate (Total)	35.880	µg
Cobalamin (Vitamin B12)	0.000	µg
Biotin	0.458	µg
Pantothenic Acid	0.261	mg
Vitamin K	11.137	µg
Phosphorus	68.560	mg
Magnesium	20.763	mg
Zinc	0.368	mg
Copper	0.066	mg
Manganese	0.199	mg
Selenium	0.260	µg
Chromium	0.005	mg
Molybdenum	1.317	µg

Recipe Tidbit:

Many different vegetables can be used for this recipe. It is easy to roast most vegetables; even broccoli and cauliflower work.

Vegetables are rich in dietary fiber. Fiber can help facilitate better bowel movements by adding bulk and weight to stools. It can also help maintain balanced blood sugar levels and is therefore especially helpful for diabetics.

BLANCHED GREEN BEANS WITH SALT

INGREDIENTS

1 pound green beans, trimmed

salt to taste

Steam green beans in about ½ inch of water until crisp-tender, around 5 minutes. Remove from heat. Sprinkle with salt; immediately place beans in a glass container and chill in refrigerator. Serve chilled.

Serves 4.

Recipe Tidbit:

You can use this simple technique for many vegetables, such as yellow beans, asparagus, broccoli, and others. It saves time if you want to make food ahead of time for a party or potluck.

Green beans are high in vitamin C, which is an important antioxidant. It is used by the body to support the immune response against infections. It speeds the healing of cuts, bruises, and injuries. It also helps to decrease blood pressure and to prevent heart disease and stroke.

Macronutrients		
Kilocalories	30.935	kcal
Protein	1.826	g
Carbohydrate	6.955	g
Fat, Total	0.220	g
Alcohol	0.000	g
Cholesterol	0.000	mg
Saturated Fat	0.050	g
Monounsaturated Fat	0.010	g
Polyunsaturated Fat	0.113	g
Trans Fatty Acid		g
Dietary Fiber, Total	2.694	g
Sugar, Total	3.253	g

Percentage of Kcals	
Protein	19.7%
Carbohydrate	75.0%
Fat, total	5.3%
Alcohol	0.0%

Vitamins & Minerals		
Sodium	151.031	mg
Potassium	189.532	mg
Vitamin A (RE)	61.970	RE
Vitamin C	9.131	mg
Calcium	35.166	mg
Iron	0.978	mg
Vitamin D (ug)	0.000	µg
Thiamin	0.065	mg
Riboflavin	0.093	mg
Niacin	0.623	mg
Pyridoxine (Vitamin B6)	0.120	mg
Folate (Total)	21.405	µg
Cobalamin (Vitamin B12)	0.000	µg
Pantothenic Acid	0.225	mg
Vitamin K	14.370	µg
Phosphorus	34.128	mg
Magnesium	23.704	mg
Zinc	0.228	mg
Copper	0.066	mg
Manganese	0.216	mg
Selenium	0.599	µg

SQUISHY CARROTS

INGREDIENTS

1 pound carrots, peeled and cut
into small sticks

Steam carrots in about ½ inch
of water over medium heat until
cooked to desired consistency. Cool
and store in the refrigerator. Snack
generously.

Serves 6.

Recipe Tidbit:

My mother-in-law, Alice Black,
steamed carrots for her dogs as
treats. My younger daughter fell in
love with them and started asking
for "squishy carrots." The glycemic
index of steamed carrots is a little
higher than that of raw carrots, but
these still provide a great alternative
to reaching for that cookie.

Macronutrients

Kilocalories	30.995	kcal
Trans Fatty Acid		g
Sugar, Total		g
Protein	0.703	g
Carbohydrate	7.242	g
Fat, Total	0.181	g
Alcohol	0.000	g
Cholesterol	0.000	mg
Saturated Fat	0.028	g
Monounsaturated Fat	0.011	g
Polyunsaturated Fat	0.088	g
Trans Fatty Acid	0.000	g
Dietary Fiber, Total	2.117	g
Sugar, Total	3.583	g

Percentage of Kcals

Protein	8.4%
Carbohydrate	86.7%
Fat, total	4.9%
Alcohol	0.0%

Vitamins & Minerals

Sodium	52.163	mg
Potassium	241.916	mg
Vitamin A (RE)	1136.656	RE
Vitamin C	3.345	mg
Calcium	24.948	mg
Iron	0.227	mg
Vitamin D (ug)	0.000	µg
Thiamin	0.045	mg
Riboflavin	0.042	mg
Niacin	0.706	mg
Pyridoxine (Vitamin B6)	0.099	mg
Folate (Total)	11.491	µg
Cobalamin (Vitamin B12)	0.000	µg
Biotin	2.268	µg
Pantothenic Acid	0.206	mg
Vitamin K	9.979	µg
Phosphorus	26.460	mg
Magnesium	9.072	mg
Zinc	0.181	mg
Copper	0.034	mg
Manganese	0.108	mg
Selenium	0.076	µg
Chromium	0.006	mg
Molybdenum	6.531	µg

FLAXSEED-OIL MAYONNAISE

INGREDIENTS

2 large egg yolks, raw

2 tablespoons lemon juice

1 cup cold flaxseed oil

1 teaspoon salt

pinch white pepper

pinch mustard powder

Macronutrients		
Kilocalories	107.357	kcal
Protein	0.302	g
Carbohydrate	0.175	g
Fat, Total	11.929	g
Alcohol	0.000	g
Cholesterol	19.416	mg
Saturated Fat	1.200	g
Monounsaturated Fat	2.322	g
Polyunsaturated Fat	7.846	g
Trans Fatty Acid	0.011	g
Dietary Fiber, Total	0.005	g
Sugar, Total	0.050	g

Percentage of Kcals	
Protein	1.1%
Carbohydrate	0.6%
Fat, total	98.3%
Alcohol	0.0%

Vitamins & Minerals		
Sodium	123.269	mg
Potassium	3.629	mg
Vitamin A (RE)	7.752	RE
Vitamin C	0.621	mg
Calcium	2.595	mg
Iron	0.051	mg
Vitamin D (ug)	0.097	µg
Thiamin	0.004	mg
Riboflavin	0.010	mg
Niacin	0.002	mg
Pyridoxine (Vitamin B6)	0.007	mg
Folate (Total)	2.934	µg
Cobalamin (Vitamin B12)	0.035	µg
Biotin	0.798	µg
Pantothenic Acid	0.056	mg
Vitamin K	1.078	µg
Phosphorus	7.222	mg
Magnesium	0.189	mg
Zinc	0.050	mg
Copper	0.002	mg
Manganese	0.001	mg
Selenium	1.004	µg

Using a handheld mixer or whisk, blend the raw egg yolks and lemon juice in a large bowl. Continue blending as you add flaxseed oil very gradually—drops at a time—until about a quarter of the oil has been added. Proceed to adding tablespoons of the oil at a time. The mixture will develop the consistency of mayonnaise. After all the oil has been added, add the mustard powder, salt, and pepper, and blend until just combined. Transfer to an airtight glass container, and store in the refrigerator.

Serving size: 1 tablespoon

Servings per jar: 16

Recipe Tidbit:

Flax-oil mayo will last about four to seven days in the refrigerator.

GREEN OLIVE TAPENADE

INGREDIENTS

1 bunch radishes, cleaned and
sliced thin

2 cucumbers, ends removed and
sliced thin

1 15-ounce jar sliced green olives

2 cloves garlic, minced

2 tablespoons olive oil

1 teaspoon anchovy paste

1 teaspoon lemon juice

1 teaspoon fresh parsley, minced

pinch cayenne pepper

pinch black pepper

Macronutrients		
Kilocalories	242.229	kcal
Protein	2.420	g
Carbohydrate	10.379	g
Fat, Total	23.353	g
Alcohol	0.000	g
Cholesterol	0.000	mg
Saturated Fat	3.149	g
Monounsaturated Fat	16.963	g
Polyunsaturated Fat	2.156	g
Trans Fatty Acid	0.000	g
Dietary Fiber, Total	4.415	g
Sugar, Total	3.269	g
Percentage of Kcals		
Protein	3.7%	
Carbohydrate	15.9%	
Fat, total	80.4%	
Alcohol	0.0%	
Vitamins & Minerals		
Sodium	1667.916	mg
Potassium	294.509	mg
Vitamin A (RE)	60.556	RE
Vitamin C	6.594	mg
Calcium	87.845	mg
Iron	1.278	mg
Vitamin D (ug)	0.000	µg
Vitamin E (mg)	0.011	mg
Thiamin	0.068	mg
Riboflavin	0.064	mg
Niacin	0.484	mg
Pyridoxine (Vitamin B6)	0.117	mg
Folate (Total)	16.192	µg
Cobalamin (Vitamin B12)	0.000	µg
Pantothenic Acid	0.437	mg
Vitamin K	35.540	µg
Phosphorus	48.178	mg
Magnesium	32.956	mg
Zinc	0.409	mg
Copper	0.205	mg
Manganese	0.149	mg
Selenium	1.663	µg

Place all ingredients except the radishes and cucumbers in a food processor, and process until coarsely chopped. Serve the tapenade on slices of cucumber and radish. Or you can eat it with seed crackers (page 68).

Serves 4.

Recipe Tidbit:

You can process longer for a smoother spread, but I like my tapenade chunky.

SAVORY SAUTÉED CELERY

INGREDIENTS

2 cloves garlic, minced

3 tablespoons butter, divided

1 large bunch celery, julienned
  into 1-inch pieces

celery leaves from the bunch,
  washed, chopped

salt and pepper to taste

Sauté the garlic in 1 tablespoon of butter over medium heat for 3 minutes. Add celery and the remaining butter, and sauté until celery begins to turn brown. Add the celery leaves and sauté a few more minutes. Season with salt and pepper and serve warm.

Serves 4.

Macronutrients

Kilocalories	97.796	kcal
Protein	1.014	g
Carbohydrate	4.066	g
Fat, Total	8.850	g
Alcohol	0.000	g
Cholesterol	22.898	mg
Saturated Fat	5.522	g
Monounsaturated Fat	2.277	g
Polyunsaturated Fat	0.423	g
Trans Fatty Acid	0.349	g
Dietary Fiber, Total	1.952	g
Sugar, Total	1.629	g

Percentage of Kcals

Protein	4.1%
Carbohydrate	16.3%
Fat, total	79.7%
Alcohol	0.0%

Vitamins & Minerals

Sodium	164.735	mg
Potassium	320.571	mg
Vitamin A (RE)	133.745	RE
Vitamin C	4.188	mg
Calcium	53.271	mg
Iron	0.268	mg
Vitamin D (ug)	0.160	µg
Vitamin E (mg)	0.248	mg
Thiamin	0.029	mg
Riboflavin	0.074	mg
Niacin	0.399	mg
Pyridoxine (Vitamin B6)	0.108	mg
Folate (Total)	43.565	µg
Cobalamin (Vitamin B12)	0.018	µg
Biotin	0.120	µg
Pantothenic Acid	0.316	mg
Vitamin K	35.931	µg
Phosphorus	33.651	mg
Magnesium	13.788	mg
Zinc	0.183	mg
Copper	0.046	mg
Manganese	0.149	mg
Selenium	0.800	µg
Chromium	0.012	mg
Molybdenum	2.001	µg

BALSAMIC HUMMUS WITH YELLOW-BEET "CHIPS"

INGREDIENTS

3 tablespoons tahini

3 tablespoons fresh lemon juice

¼ cup water

2 tablespoons olive oil, divided

1 garlic clove

1 15-ounce can navy beans, drained,
   or 1½ cups cooked navy beans

½ teaspoon salt

1–2 tablespoons good-quality
   balsamic vinegar

3 large yellow beets, peeled and
   sliced into "chips"

Macronutrients		
Kilocalories	278.839	kcal
Protein	11.001	g
Carbohydrate	31.187	g
Fat, Total	13.279	g
Alcohol	0.000	g
Cholesterol	0.000	mg
Saturated Fat	1.903	g
Monounsaturated Fat	7.237	g
Polyunsaturated Fat	3.560	g
Trans Fatty Acid	0.000	g
Dietary Fiber, Total	7.688	g
Sugar, Total	5.363	g
Percentage of Kcals		
Protein	15.3%	
Carbohydrate	43.3%	
Fat, total	41.5%	
Alcohol	0.0%	
Vitamins & Minerals		
Sodium	820.321	mg
Potassium	563.595	mg
Vitamin A (RE)	2.792	RE
Vitamin C	4.483	mg
Calcium	78.168	mg
Iron	3.028	mg
Vitamin D (ug)	0.000	µg
Vitamin E (mg)	0.000	mg
Thiamin	0.368	mg
Riboflavin	0.116	mg
Niacin	1.382	mg
Pyridoxine (Vitamin B6)	0.177	mg
Folate (Total)	143.995	µg
Cobalamin (Vitamin B12)	0.000	µg
Pantothenic Acid	0.283	mg
Vitamin K	7.282	µg
Phosphorus	257.829	mg
Magnesium	75.967	mg
Zinc	1.563	mg
Copper	0.454	mg
Manganese	0.614	mg
Selenium	10.574	µg

In a food processor or high-powered blender, blend together the tahini, lemon juice, water, 1 tablespoon of the olive oil, and garlic until smooth. Add the navy beans, salt, and 1 tablespoon of the vinegar, and blend to your desired consistency (chunky or smooth). Taste, and add more vinegar if you wish. I like using a full 2 tablespoons of vinegar because I like my hummus tangy.

Garnish with the remaining olive oil when serving. Serve with yellow beets for dipping.

Serves 4.

Recipe Tidbit:

It is very easy to replace chips and crackers with vegetables. Any vegetable that can be cut into a shape like a chip can be used like a chip. Yellow beets are delicious raw, and they don't stain your hands the way red beets do.

BASIL PESTO

INGREDIENTS

4 cups fresh basil leaves, washed
and patted dry

½ cup extra-virgin olive oil

3–4 cloves garlic

⅓ cup pine nuts

½ cup pecorino Romano cheese
(optional)

¼ teaspoon salt

¼ teaspoon pepper (optional)

Process all ingredients in a food
processor until smooth.

Serves 4.

Macronutrients		
Kilocalories	328.874	kcal
Protein	3.046	g
Carbohydrate	3.365	g
Fat, Total	35.114	g
Alcohol	0.000	g
Cholesterol	0.000	mg
Saturated Fat	4.309	g
Monounsaturated Fat	21.886	g
Polyunsaturated Fat	6.915	g
Trans Fatty Acid		g
Dietary Fiber, Total	1.149	g
Sugar, Total	0.561	g

Percentage of Kcals	
Protein	3.6%
Carbohydrate	3.9%
Fat, total	92.5%
Alcohol	0.0%

Vitamins & Minerals		
Sodium	148.190	mg
Potassium	202.743	mg
Vitamin A (RE)	223.936	RE
Vitamin C	8.423	mg
Calcium	81.285	mg
Iron	2.168	mg
Vitamin D (ug)	0.000	µg
Thiamin	0.061	mg
Riboflavin	0.061	mg
Niacin	0.901	mg
Pyridoxine (Vitamin B6)	0.104	mg
Folate (Total)	32.783	µg
Cobalamin (Vitamin B12)	0.000	µg
Pantothenic Acid	0.138	mg
Vitamin K	198.275	µg
Phosphorus	93.045	mg
Magnesium	56.445	mg
Zinc	1.109	mg
Copper	0.322	mg
Manganese	1.533	mg
Selenium	0.527	µg

Recipe Tidbit:

Basil isn't the only herb that makes a
delicious pesto; you can use cilantro,
spinach, or parsley. You could even try a combination of two different herbs
for variety. For example, use 2 cups basil with 2 cups spinach. I have made a
chive pesto that turned out deliciously spicy.

Try this recipe both with and without the cheese. I use about half the
amount of cheese called for in other pesto recipes.

Pine nuts give lubrication to the lungs and intestines. They are a great
source of protein, can aid in coughs, and help decrease constipation. Or
you could substitute different nuts, such as walnuts or pecans, each of
which affords nutritional benefits of its own.

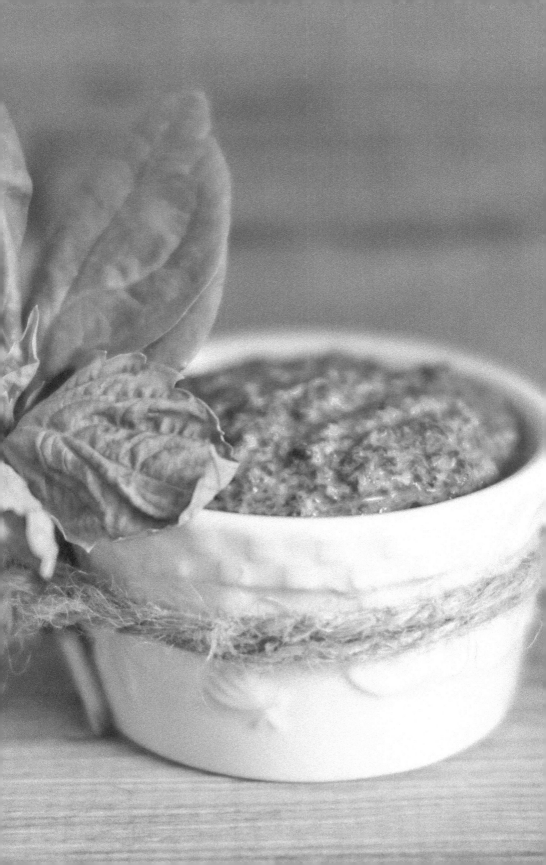

LEMON ASPARAGUS WITH DILL

INGREDIENTS

2 bunches asparagus (about 1
pound)

2 tablespoons fresh lemon juice
(juice from 1 medium lemon)

3 tablespoons olive oil

2 teaspoons fresh dill

½ teaspoon salt

¼ teaspoon black pepper

Macronutrients		
Kilocalories	114.232	kcal
Protein	2.538	g
Carbohydrate	5.016	g
Fat, Total	10.285	g
Alcohol	0.000	g
Cholesterol	0.000	mg
Saturated Fat	1.448	g
Monounsaturated Fat	7.389	g
Polyunsaturated Fat	1.125	g
Trans Fatty Acid	0.000	g
Dietary Fiber, Total	2.439	g
Sugar, Total	2.325	g
Percentage of Kcals		
Protein	8.3%	
Carbohydrate	16.3%	
Fat, total	75.4%	
Alcohol	0.0%	
Vitamins & Minerals		
Sodium	293.315	mg
Potassium	239.512	mg
Vitamin A (RE)	82.248	RE
Vitamin C	8.428	mg
Calcium	28.730	mg
Iron	2.511	mg
Vitamin D (ug)	0.000	µg
Thiamin	0.148	mg
Riboflavin	0.154	mg
Niacin	1.063	mg
Pyridoxine (Vitamin B6)	0.097	mg
Folate (Total)	51.809	µg
Cobalamin (Vitamin B12)	0.000	µg
Pantothenic Acid	0.323	mg
Vitamin K	53.484	µg
Phosphorus	59.846	mg
Magnesium	16.617	mg
Zinc	0.619	mg
Copper	0.218	mg
Manganese	0.199	mg
Selenium	2.623	µg
Chromium	0.001	mg

Wash the asparagus, cut off the ends, and steam until the stems are cooked but still a little firm. In a bowl, mix together lemon juice, olive oil, dill, salt, and pepper. Arrange the asparagus on a serving dish, and drizzle with the lemon juice mixture. Serve immediately.

Serves 4.

Recipe Tidbit:

You could substitute green beans for the asparagus. You can top the dish with freshly grated pecorino or Romano cheese.

SOAKED QUINOA

INGREDIENTS

1 cup quinoa

1 tablespoon apple cider vinegar or
whey

2 cups filtered water

Combine all ingredients in a medium saucepan or rice cooker, cover, and allow to sit over night or for 12 hours during the day. After soaking, the quinoa seeds will have sprouted. When ready, transfer to the stove and bring to a boil. Reduce heat and simmer until all water has been absorbed by the quinoa, about 10–20 minutes.

Serves 4.

Recipe Tidbit:

It is best to soak grains before consuming them.

Macronutrients		
Kilocalories	157.182	kcal
Protein	6.001	g
Carbohydrate	27.303	g
Fat, Total	2.580	g
Alcohol	0.000	g
Cholesterol	0.000	mg
Saturated Fat	0.300	g
Monounsaturated Fat	0.686	g
Polyunsaturated Fat	1.399	g
Trans Fatty Acid	0.000	g
Dietary Fiber, Total	2.975	g
Sugar, Total	0.015	g

Percentage of Kcals	
Protein	15.3%
Carbohydrate	69.8%
Fat, total	14.8%
Alcohol	0.0%

Vitamins & Minerals		
Sodium	5.866	mg
Potassium	243.179	mg
Vitamin A (RE)	0.595	RE
Vitamin C	0.000	mg
Calcium	23.791	mg
Iron	1.950	mg
Vitamin D (ug)	0.000	µg
Thiamin	0.153	mg
Riboflavin	0.135	mg
Niacin	0.646	mg
Pyridoxine (Vitamin B6)	0.207	mg
Folate (Total)	78.200	µg
Cobalamin (Vitamin B12)	0.000	µg
Pantothenic Acid	0.328	mg
Vitamin K	0.000	µg
Phosphorus	194.523	mg
Magnesium	85.096	mg
Zinc	1.319	mg
Copper	0.262	mg
Manganese	0.873	mg
Selenium	3.616	µg

SOAKED BROWN RICE

INGREDIENTS

1 cup brown rice, short or long grain

1 tablespoon apple cider vinegar
   or whey

2 cups filtered water

Combine all ingredients in a medium saucepan or rice cooker, cover, and allow to sit over night or for 12 hours during the day. When ready, transfer to the stove and bring to a boil. Reduce heat and simmer until all water has been absorbed by the rice, about 45 minutes.

Serves 4.

Recipe Tidbit:
   It is best to soak grains before consuming them.

Macronutrients		
Kilocalories	172.121	kcal
Protein	3.687	g
Carbohydrate	35.975	g
Fat, Total	1.354	g
Alcohol	0.000	g
Cholesterol	0.000	mg
Saturated Fat	0.271	g
Monounsaturated Fat	0.488	g
Polyunsaturated Fat	0.484	g
Trans Fatty Acid		g
Dietary Fiber, Total	1.641	g
Sugar, Total	0.618	g

Percentage of Kcals	
Protein	8.6%
Carbohydrate	84.2%
Fat, total	7.1%
Alcohol	0.0%

Vitamins & Minerals		
Sodium	7.290	mg
Potassium	110.628	mg
Vitamin A (RE)	0.138	RE
Vitamin C	0.498	mg
Calcium	14.358	mg
Iron	0.685	mg
Vitamin D (ug)	0.000	µg
Thiamin	0.187	mg
Riboflavin	0.043	mg
Niacin	2.366	mg
Pyridoxine (Vitamin B6)	0.238	mg
Folate (Total)	9.775	µg
Cobalamin (Vitamin B12)	0.000	µg
Pantothenic Acid	0.695	mg
Vitamin K	0.959	µg
Phosphorus	154.317	mg
Magnesium	67.599	mg
Zinc	0.937	mg
Copper	0.139	mg
Manganese	1.732	mg
Selenium	10.842	µg

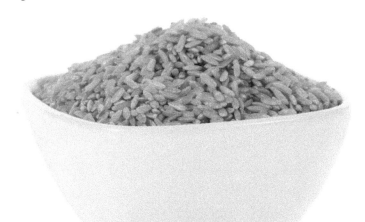

Chapter 3
SALADS

CHICKEN SALAD

INGREDIENTS

1 pound chicken breasts

½ small onion, minced

1 cup celery, diced

1 cup sunflower seeds

½ cup mayonnaise

2 teaspoons fresh tarragon, minced

½ teaspoon salt

Preheat oven to 350°F. Pour 1–2 inches of water into a deep baking dish. Add chicken breasts, cover, and bake for 12–15 minutes, until chicken is tender but thoroughly cooked through. Remove from oven and allow to cool. While the chicken is cooling, combine remaining ingredients in a medium-sized mixing bowl. After the chicken has cooled, cut it into cubes, add to the remaining ingredients, and mix to combine.

Serve chilled over salad greens or with seed crackers.

Serves 4.

Recipe Tidbit:

You can substitute other seasonings for the tarragon, such as curry powder or dill.

Macronutrients		
Kilocalories	542.268	kcal
Trans Fatty Acid		g
Sugar, Total		g
Protein	33.626	g
Carbohydrate	9.391	g
Fat, Total	42.017	g
Alcohol	0.000	g
Cholesterol	94.189	mg
Saturated Fat	5.427	g
Monounsaturated Fat	12.017	g
Polyunsaturated Fat	21.123	g
Trans Fatty Acid	0.060	g
Dietary Fiber, Total	3.734	g
Sugar, Total	2.022	g

Percentage of Kcals	
Protein	24.4%
Carbohydrate	6.8%
Fat, total	68.7%
Alcohol	0.0%

Vitamins & Minerals		
Sodium	530.868	mg
Potassium	632.106	mg
Vitamin A (RE)	22.886	RE
Vitamin C	2.329	mg
Calcium	51.241	mg
Iron	2.407	mg
Vitamin D (ug)	0.055	µg
Thiamin	0.624	mg
Riboflavin	0.332	mg
Niacin	11.806	mg
Pyridoxine (Vitamin B6)	1.257	mg
Folate (Total)	100.926	µg
Cobalamin (Vitamin B12)	0.188	µg
Biotin	3.503	µg
Pantothenic Acid	2.228	mg
Vitamin K	52.668	µg
Phosphorus	447.233	mg
Magnesium	145.885	mg
Zinc	2.677	mg
Copper	0.708	mg
Manganese	0.761	mg
Selenium	45.738	µg
Chromium	0.006	mg
Molybdenum	0.500	µg

COLESLAW

INGREDIENTS

½ head purple cabbage, shredded

½ head white cabbage, shredded

1 cup kale, chopped fine

2 carrots, grated

1 cup pumpkin seeds

¾ cup mayonnaise

½ cup red wine vinegar

2 teaspoons poppy seeds

½ teaspoon salt

½ teaspoon black pepper

Combine all ingredients in a large mixing bowl, cover, and transfer to the refrigerator to allow flavors to mingle for 12 hours before serving. Serve chilled. Serves 6.

Macronutrients		
Kilocalories	371.398	kcal
Trans Fatty Acid		g
Sugar, Total		g
Protein	9.885	g
Carbohydrate	8.634	g
Fat, Total	33.402	g
Alcohol	0.000	g
Cholesterol	11.592	mg
Saturated Fat	5.368	g
Monounsaturated Fat	8.562	g
Polyunsaturated Fat	18.057	g
Trans Fatty Acid	0.066	g
Dietary Fiber, Total	2.942	g
Sugar, Total	3.495	g

Percentage of Kcals	
Protein	10.6%
Carbohydrate	9.2%
Fat, total	80.2%
Alcohol	0.0%

Vitamins & Minerals		
Sodium	397.596	mg
Potassium	497.883	mg
Vitamin A (RE)	457.702	RE
Vitamin C	47.715	mg
Calcium	106.607	mg
Iron	3.499	mg
Vitamin D (ug)	0.055	µg
Vitamin E (mg)	0.070	mg
Thiamin	0.206	mg
Riboflavin	0.087	mg
Niacin	1.731	mg
Pyridoxine (Vitamin B6)	0.164	mg
Folate (Total)	48.554	µg
Cobalamin (Vitamin B12)	0.033	µg
Biotin	3.965	µg
Pantothenic Acid	0.371	mg
Vitamin K	149.340	µg
Phosphorus	415.263	mg
Magnesium	157.045	mg
Zinc	2.319	mg
Copper	0.544	mg
Manganese	1.439	mg
Selenium	3.305	µg
Chromium	0.002	mg
Molybdenum	1.757	µg

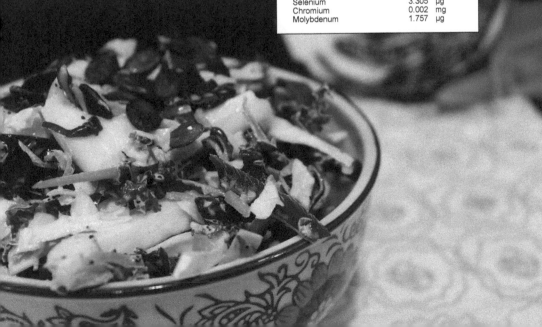

PICTURESQUE SALAD

INGREDIENTS

4 cups mixed greens

1 broccoli crown, chopped

1 avocado, diced

1 14.5-ounce can medium pitted
black olives (packed only in water
and salt)

2 hard-boiled eggs, cut into chunks

1 large tomato, chopped

1 cup crimini mushrooms, stems
removed and chopped

1 orange bell pepper, chopped

For the dressing:

⅓ cup olive oil

¼ cup red wine vinegar

1 tablespoon mustard

pinch salt

pinch pepper

Macronutrients		
Kilocalories	423.108	kcal
Trans Fatty Acid		g
Sugar, Total		g
Protein	8.034	g
Carbohydrate	19.416	g
Fat, Total	37.350	g
Alcohol	0.000	g
Cholesterol	93.250	mg
Saturated Fat	5.537	g
Monounsaturated Fat	25.629	g
Polyunsaturated Fat	3.977	g
Trans Fatty Acid	0.000	g
Dietary Fiber, Total	8.521	g
Sugar, Total	3.848	g

Percentage of Kcals	
Protein	7.2%
Carbohydrate	17.4%
Fat, total	75.4%
Alcohol	0.0%

Vitamins & Minerals		
Sodium	857.881	mg
Potassium	766.888	mg
Vitamin A (RE)	199.974	RE
Vitamin C	137.541	mg
Calcium	165.417	mg
Iron	5.121	mg
Vitamin D (ug)	0.574	µg
Vitamin E (mg)	0.363	mg
Thiamin	0.153	mg
Riboflavin	0.392	mg
Niacin	2.645	mg
Pyridoxine (Vitamin B6)	0.366	mg
Folate (Total)	131.053	µg
Cobalamin (Vitamin B12)	0.302	µg
Biotin	6.772	µg
Pantothenic Acid	1.776	mg
Vitamin K	113.717	µg
Phosphorus	160.012	mg
Magnesium	46.693	mg
Zinc	1.534	mg
Copper	0.585	mg
Manganese	0.420	mg
Selenium	17.532	µg
Chromium	0.020	mg
Molybdenum	0.338	µg

Whisk together vinegar, mustard, salt, and pepper. Gradually whisk in olive oil, ½ teaspoon or so at a time, blending thoroughly after each addition to emulsify the mixture. Set dressing aside to allow flavors to mingle.

Layer the greens on the bottoms of 4 individual serving bowls, and top with a straight line of each ingredient across the salad, paying special attention to the arrangement of colors. I arrange the ingredients to make a rainbow: tomatoes, orange pepper, hard-boiled eggs, broccoli, avocado, black olives, mushrooms. This makes an amazingly pretty salad to serve to guests. Serve with dressing on the side.

Serves 4.

Recipe Tidbit:
    See the recipe for perfect hard-boiled eggs on page 62.

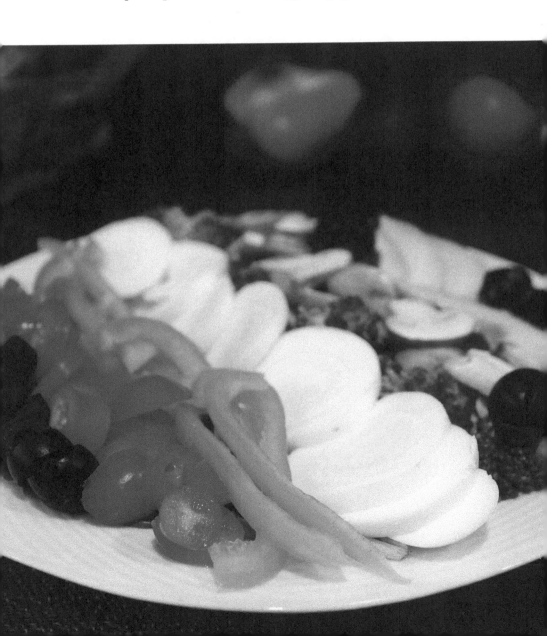

EASY SALMON SALAD

INGREDIENTS

2 7-ounce cans salmon, wild
  caught, boneless, skinless

½ cup mayonnaise

2 carrots, minced

2 stalks celery, minced

1 teaspoon dried dill

½ teaspoon salt

In a medium mixing bowl, combine all ingredients. Serve chilled over salad greens or with seed crackers.

Serves 4.

Macronutrients		
Kilocalories	291.518	kcal
Trans Fatty Acid		g
Sugar, Total		g
Protein	19.987	g
Carbohydrate	3.813	g
Fat, Total	22.527	g
Alcohol	0.000	g
Cholesterol	46.592	mg
Saturated Fat	3.250	g
Monounsaturated Fat	4.927	g
Polyunsaturated Fat	12.771	g
Trans Fatty Acid	0.052	g
Dietary Fiber, Total	1.208	g
Sugar, Total	1.871	g

Percentage of Kcals	
Protein	26.8%
Carbohydrate	5.1%
Fat, total	68.0%
Alcohol	0.0%

Vitamins & Minerals		
Sodium	766.010	mg
Potassium	163.450	mg
Vitamin A (RE)	523.564	RE
Vitamin C	2.545	mg
Calcium	24.913	mg
Iron	0.314	mg
Vitamin D (ug)	0.055	µg
Thiamin	0.028	mg
Riboflavin	0.035	mg
Niacin	0.371	mg
Pyridoxine (Vitamin B6)	0.063	mg
Folate (Total)	14.750	µg
Cobalamin (Vitamin B12)	0.033	µg
Biotin	4.255	µg
Pantothenic Acid	0.181	mg
Vitamin K	54.874	µg
Phosphorus	22.629	mg
Magnesium	7.271	mg
Zinc	0.150	mg
Copper	0.027	mg
Manganese	0.077	mg
Selenium	0.746	µg
Chromium	0.005	mg
Molybdenum	2.968	µg

BALSAMIC CHICKEN SALAD WITH PEPPERS

INGREDIENTS

4 cups romaine lettuce, chopped

1 red bell pepper, chopped large

2 cups cubed baked chicken breast, chilled

1 cup cottage cheese

For the dressing:

½ cup olive oil

⅓ cup balsamic vinegar

1 teaspoon dried basil

½ teaspoon salt

Whisk together vinegar, basil, and salt. Gradually whisk in olive oil, ½ teaspoon or so at a time, blending thoroughly after each addition to emulsify the mixture. Set dressing aside to allow flavors to mingle.

In 4 individual serving bowls, layer the salad ingredients in the following order: romaine on the bottom, then peppers, chicken, and cottage cheese. Top with dressing, and enjoy.

Serves 4.

Macronutrients		
Kilocalories	442.749	kcal
Trans Fatty Acid		g
Sugar, Total		g
Protein	28.598	g
Carbohydrate	11.392	g
Fat, Total	31.026	g
Alcohol	0.000	g
Cholesterol	66.280	mg
Saturated Fat	5.167	g
Monounsaturated Fat	20.870	g
Polyunsaturated Fat	3.525	g
Trans Fatty Acid	0.000	g
Dietary Fiber, Total	1.744	g
Sugar, Total	4.075	g

Percentage of Kcals	
Protein	26.0%
Carbohydrate	10.4%
Fat, total	63.6%
Alcohol	0.0%

Vitamins & Minerals		
Sodium	522.261	mg
Potassium	438.224	mg
Vitamin A (RE)	522.754	RE
Vitamin C	39.874	mg
Calcium	99.098	mg
Iron	1.853	mg
Vitamin D (ug)	0.070	µg
Thiamin	0.110	mg
Riboflavin	0.283	mg
Niacin	10.112	mg
Pyridoxine (Vitamin B6)	0.578	mg
Folate (Total)	86.010	µg
Cobalamin (Vitamin B12)	0.504	µg
Biotin	2.540	µg
Pantothenic Acid	1.136	mg
Vitamin K	72.098	µg
Phosphorus	267.145	mg
Magnesium	38.031	mg
Zinc	1.196	mg
Copper	0.088	mg
Manganese	0.162	mg
Selenium	26.273	µg
Chromium	0.027	mg
Molybdenum	3.439	µg

SWEET POTATO KALE SALAD

INGREDIENTS

4 cups kale, stems removed and
   chopped
2 sweet potatoes, cooked, cubed,
   and chilled
1 cup walnuts, chopped or whole

For the dressing:
4 tablespoons water
1 tablespoon tahini
1 tablespoon olive oil
1 tablespoon lemon juice
1 tablespoon stone-ground mustard
2 garlic cloves, minced
¼ teaspoon salt, or to taste

In a large mixing bowl, whisk together dressing ingredients, blending thoroughly. Add salad ingredients, and stir to combine. Serve chilled.

Serves 4.

Macronutrients		
Kilocalories	335.134	kcal
Trans Fatty Acid		g
Sugar, Total		g
Protein	9.104	g
Carbohydrate	24.516	g
Fat, Total	25.109	g
Alcohol	0.000	g
Cholesterol	0.000	mg
Saturated Fat	2.612	g
Monounsaturated Fat	5.862	g
Polyunsaturated Fat	15.265	g
Trans Fatty Acid	0.000	g
Dietary Fiber, Total	6.541	g
Sugar, Total	5.106	g

Percentage of Kcals	
Protein	10.1%
Carbohydrate	27.2%
Fat, total	62.7%
Alcohol	0.0%

Vitamins & Minerals		
Sodium	258.005	mg
Potassium	704.379	mg
Vitamin A (RE)	1592.357	RE
Vitamin C	84.441	mg
Calcium	157.464	mg
Iron	2.447	mg
Vitamin D (ug)	0.000	µg
Thiamin	0.288	mg
Riboflavin	0.177	mg
Niacin	1.587	mg
Pyridoxine (Vitamin B6)	0.500	mg
Folate (Total)	134.768	µg
Cobalamin (Vitamin B12)	0.000	µg
Biotin	11.100	µg
Pantothenic Acid	0.762	mg
Vitamin K	476.233	µg
Phosphorus	225.620	mg
Magnesium	98.273	mg
Zinc	1.667	mg
Copper	1.633	mg
Manganese	1.634	mg
Selenium	3.933	µg

Recipe Tidbit:

   Tahini, or sesame-seed paste, can be expensive. If you don't want to purchase tahini, you can simply grind 2 tablespoons of roasted sesame seeds in the blender with 1 tablespoon of water. Roast raw sesame seeds by cooking them in a skillet over medium heat, tossing constantly until they begin to brown. Immediately remove them from the heat to avoid burning.

   This is another recipe that readily lends itself to substitutions. Use these recipes as templates for generating your own ideas.

BACON BROCCOLI SALAD

INGREDIENTS

4 crowns broccoli, chopped

1 cup kale, stems removed, chopped

1 red onion, chopped

1 pound turkey bacon

1 cup sunflower seeds

1 pint cherry tomatoes, halved

For the dressing:

½ cup mayonnaise

½ cup red wine vinegar

½ teaspoon salt

Macronutrients		
Kilocalories	933.204	kcal
Trans Fatty Acid		g
Sugar, Total		g
Protein	48.156	g
Carbohydrate	27.073	g
Fat, Total	72.020	g
Alcohol	0.000	g
Cholesterol	122.724	mg
Saturated Fat	14.422	g
Monounsaturated Fat	23.796	g
Polyunsaturated Fat	28.683	g
Trans Fatty Acid	0.052	g
Dietary Fiber, Total	8.898	g
Sugar, Total	8.291	g
Percentage of Kcals		
Protein	20.3%	
Carbohydrate	11.4%	
Fat, total	68.3%	
Alcohol	0.0%	
Vitamins & Minerals		
Sodium	3141.356	mg
Potassium	1641.563	mg
Vitamin A (RE)	355.846	RE
Vitamin C	208.946	mg
Calcium	168.819	mg
Iron	6.451	mg
Vitamin D (ug)	0.509	µg
Vitamin E (mg)	1.038	mg
Thiamin	0.815	mg
Riboflavin	0.681	mg
Niacin	9.216	mg
Pyridoxine (Vitamin B6)	1.365	mg
Folate (Total)	251.267	µg
Cobalamin (Vitamin B12)	0.441	µg
Biotin	4.596	µg
Pantothenic Acid	1.725	mg
Vitamin K	348.064	µg
Phosphorus	936.455	mg
Magnesium	209.567	mg
Zinc	6.344	mg
Copper	1.229	mg
Manganese	1.296	mg
Selenium	53.811	µg
Chromium	0.034	mg

Preheat broiler. Arrange bacon in a single layer on a broiling pan, and place under the broiler until bacon is cooked and crispy, but not over-cooked, about 4–5 minutes. Remove bacon from oven and transfer onto a paper towel. If you would like crisper bacon, leave it on the baking sheet for a bit after removing it from the oven; it will continue to cook. Set bacon aside until it is cool enough to cut into 1-inch pieces.

While the bacon is cooking, whisk together the dressing ingredients, and set aside. Prepare the other ingredients for the salad, and combine in a large mixing bowl. Add the chilled or warm bacon to the other ingredients, and toss with the salad dressing. Chill for up to 4 hours before serving.

Serves 4.

ROMAINE GREEK SALAD

INGREDIENTS

3 romaine hearts, washed and
chopped

2 cups chopped cucumber

2 cups chopped tomatoes

1 large red onion, sliced thin

¾ cup feta cheese, crumbled

¾ cup pitted kalamata olives

For the dressing:

½ cup olive oil

¼ cup red wine vinegar

2 tablespoons lemon juice

1 teaspoon dried oregano

In a large mixing bowl, whisk together vinegar, lemon juice, and oregano. Gradually whisk in olive oil, ½ teaspoon or so at a time, blending thoroughly after each addition to emulsify the mixture. Add the salad ingredients to the bowl, and toss to combine with the dressing.

Serves 8.

Macronutrients		
Kilocalories	214.696	kcal
Trans Fatty Acid		g
Sugar, Total		g
Protein	2.845	g
Carbohydrate	7.447	g
Fat, Total	19.729	g
Alcohol	0.000	g
Cholesterol	9.375	mg
Saturated Fat	3.404	g
Monounsaturated Fat	9.871	g
Polyunsaturated Fat	1.501	g
Trans Fatty Acid	0.000	g
Dietary Fiber, Total	1.568	g
Sugar, Total	2.516	g

Percentage of Kcals	
Protein	5.2%
Carbohydrate	13.6%
Fat, total	81.2%
Alcohol	0.0%

Vitamins & Minerals		
Sodium	351.194	mg
Potassium	218.301	mg
Vitamin A (RE)	227.888	RE
Vitamin C	10.133	mg
Calcium	52.046	mg
Iron	0.589	mg
Vitamin D (ug)	0.000	µg
Vitamin E (mg)	0.171	mg
Thiamin	0.044	mg
Riboflavin	0.034	mg
Niacin	0.378	mg
Pyridoxine (Vitamin B6)	0.080	mg
Folate (Total)	36.448	µg
Cobalamin (Vitamin B12)	0.000	µg
Biotin	1.206	µg
Pantothenic Acid	0.139	mg
Vitamin K	35.465	µg
Phosphorus	27.553	mg
Magnesium	13.309	mg
Zinc	0.203	mg
Copper	0.054	mg
Manganese	0.114	mg
Selenium	0.231	µg
Chromium	0.005	mg
Molybdenum	0.315	µg

BLT SALAD

INGREDIENTS

1 pound turkey bacon

1 head butter lettuce, torn into leaves

3 large tomatoes, chopped

1 near-ripe avocado, pitted and cubed

For the dressing:

¾ cup mayonnaise

¼ cup olive oil

¼ cup red wine vinegar

½ teaspoon celery seed

½ teaspoon salt

Macronutrients		
Kilocalories	915.593	kcal
Trans Fatty Acid		g
Sugar, Total		g
Protein	36.032	g
Carbohydrate	11.280	g
Fat, Total	81.614	g
Alcohol	0.000	g
Cholesterol	128.520	mg
Saturated Fat	16.868	g
Monounsaturated Fat	32.529	g
Polyunsaturated Fat	28.382	g
Trans Fatty Acid	0.077	g
Dietary Fiber, Total	3.857	g
Sugar, Total	3.147	g

Percentage of Kcals	
Protein	15.6%
Carbohydrate	4.9%
Fat, total	79.5%
Alcohol	0.0%

Vitamins & Minerals		
Sodium	3155.958	mg
Potassium	950.814	mg
Vitamin A (RE)	222.116	RE
Vitamin C	17.205	mg
Calcium	46.983	mg
Iron	3.696	mg
Vitamin D (ug)	0.536	µg
Vitamin E (mg)	0.179	mg
Thiamin	0.155	mg
Riboflavin	0.371	mg
Niacin	5.343	mg
Pyridoxine (Vitamin B6)	0.572	mg
Folate (Total)	85.630	µg
Cobalamin (Vitamin B12)	0.458	µg
Biotin	9.878	µg
Pantothenic Acid	0.703	mg
Vitamin K	131.602	µg
Phosphorus	586.536	mg
Magnesium	60.144	mg
Zinc	3.986	mg
Copper	0.301	mg
Manganese	0.257	mg
Selenium	30.619	µg
Chromium	0.033	mg
Molybdenum	0.739	µg

Preheat broiler. Arrange bacon in a single layer on a broiling pan, and place under the broiler until bacon is cooked and crispy, but not over-cooked, about 4–5 minutes. Remove bacon from oven and transfer onto a paper towel. If you would like crisper bacon, leave it on the baking sheet for a bit after removing it from the oven; it will continue to cook. Set bacon aside until it is cool enough to cut into 1-inch pieces. If you have time, transfer the cut bacon to the refrigerator so it has time to cool thoroughly.

While the bacon is cooking, prepare the dressing by whisking together all ingredients. Set aside. Prepare the salad ingredients, and combine them in a large mixing bowl. Add the bacon, and toss with the salad dressing. Serve immediately.

Serves 4.

Recipe Tidbit:

Make sure to use an avocado that is not overripe, which would be too mushy for this recipe.

KALE CAESAR SALAD

INGREDIENTS

6 cups kale, stems removed, chopped

1 large carrot, grated

½ cup coarsely grated Parmesan

For the dressing:

¾ cup mayonnaise

½ cup freshly grated Parmesan

2 garlic cloves

2 tablespoons freshly squeezed
lemon juice (from one lemon)

1 teaspoon anchovy paste

1 teaspoon Dijon mustard

¼ teaspoon salt

¼ teaspoon freshly ground black
pepper

Macronutrients		
Kilocalories	428.634	kcal
Trans Fatty Acid		g
Sugar, Total		g
Protein	10.852	g
Carbohydrate	14.379	g
Fat, Total	37.688	g
Alcohol	0.000	g
Cholesterol	34.588	mg
Saturated Fat	8.023	g
Monounsaturated Fat	8.455	g
Polyunsaturated Fat	19.143	g
Trans Fatty Acid	0.077	g
Dietary Fiber, Total	4.133	g
Sugar, Total	3.458	g

Percentage of Kcals	
Protein	9.9%
Carbohydrate	13.1%
Fat, total	77.1%
Alcohol	0.0%

Vitamins & Minerals		
Sodium	855.602	mg
Potassium	605.928	mg
Vitamin A (RE)	1291.003	RE
Vitamin C	124.919	mg
Calcium	337.039	mg
Iron	1.982	mg
Vitamin D (ug)	0.183	µg
Vitamin E (mg)	0.011	mg
Thiamin	0.135	mg
Riboflavin	0.224	mg
Niacin	1.241	mg
Pyridoxine (Vitamin B6)	0.335	mg
Folate (Total)	149.465	µg
Cobalamin (Vitamin B12)	0.330	µg
Biotin	6.038	µg
Pantothenic Acid	0.315	mg
Vitamin K	778.399	µg
Phosphorus	238.879	mg
Magnesium	57.752	mg
Zinc	1.550	mg
Copper	1.544	mg
Manganese	0.744	mg
Selenium	8.979	µg
Chromium	0.002	mg
Molybdenum	2.237	µg

Combine all dressing ingredients in a high-powered blender or food processor, and process until smooth. Toss the kale with enough dressing to lightly coat the leaves. I use about half the dressing and save the other half for the next time. Top the dressed kale with carrots and Parmesan. Serve immediately, or chill until serving.

Serves 4.

Recipe Tidbit:

Be creative with this salad. You can add white beans, tomatoes, red cabbage, seeds, radishes, or avocados.

NEEDS-NO-DRESSING SALAD

INGREDIENTS

4 cups mixed greens

4 green onions, chopped fine

1 large or 2 small tomatoes, chopped

1 large carrot, grated

1 cucumber, chopped

1 14.5-ounce can medium pitted black olives (packed only in water and salt)

1 cup roasted and salted sunflower seeds

Combine all ingredients, and enjoy.

Serves 4.

Recipe Tidbit:

Begin to enjoy salads without needing salad dressing. It has taken me a long time to develop a taste for dressing-free salads because I traditionally loved dressings. This recipe was inspired by a friend of mine who served beautiful salads that had no need for dressing.

Macronutrients		
Kilocalories	363.760	kcal
Trans Fatty Acid		g
Sugar, Total		g
Protein	10.126	g
Carbohydrate	21.491	g
Fat, Total	29.823	g
Alcohol	0.000	g
Cholesterol	0.000	mg
Saturated Fat	3.125	g
Monounsaturated Fat	14.801	g
Polyunsaturated Fat	9.398	g
Trans Fatty Acid	0.000	g
Dietary Fiber, Total	8.642	g
Sugar, Total	4.357	g
Percentage of Kcals		
Protein	10.3%	
Carbohydrate	21.8%	
Fat, total	68.0%	
Alcohol	0.0%	
Vitamins & Minerals		
Sodium	781.530	mg
Potassium	637.354	mg
Vitamin A (RE)	397.568	RE
Vitamin C	14.931	mg
Calcium	170.262	mg
Iron	6.118	mg
Vitamin D (ug)	0.000	µg
Vitamin E (mg)	0.363	mg
Thiamin	0.608	mg
Riboflavin	0.204	mg
Niacin	3.656	mg
Pyridoxine (Vitamin B6)	0.597	mg
Folate (Total)	142.777	µg
Cobalamin (Vitamin B12)	0.000	µg
Biotin	2.840	µg
Pantothenic Acid	0.883	mg
Vitamin K	94.922	µg
Phosphorus	290.273	mg
Magnesium	146.419	mg
Zinc	2.532	mg
Copper	1.027	mg
Manganese	0.964	mg
Selenium	20.336	µg
Chromium	0.015	mg
Molybdenum	1.655	µg

ARUGULA SPROUT SALAD

INGREDIENTS

6 cups arugula

2 cups enoki mushrooms

1 package mung bean sprouts

1 cup feta cheese, crumbled

For the dressing:

¾ cup mayonnaise

2 garlic cloves, minced

2 tablespoons freshly squeezed
lemon juice (from one lemon)

1 teaspoon Dijon mustard

¼ teaspoon salt

¼ teaspoon freshly ground black
pepper

½ teaspoon poppy seeds

Macronutrients		
Kilocalories	413.354	kcal
Trans Fatty Acid		g
Sugar, Total		g
Protein	8.562	g
Carbohydrate	10.124	g
Fat, Total	38.557	g
Alcohol	0.000	g
Cholesterol	42.388	mg
Saturated Fat	8.916	g
Monounsaturated Fat	7.016	g
Polyunsaturated Fat	18.765	g
Trans Fatty Acid	0.077	g
Dietary Fiber, Total	2.996	g
Sugar, Total	2.350	g
Percentage of Kcals		
Protein	8.1%	
Carbohydrate	9.6%	
Fat, total	82.3%	
Alcohol	0.0%	
Vitamins & Minerals		
Sodium	849.982	mg
Potassium	358.880	mg
Vitamin A (RE)	167.275	RE
Vitamin C	11.665	mg
Calcium	143.874	mg
Iron	1.438	mg
Vitamin D (ug)	0.133	µg
Thiamin	0.162	mg
Riboflavin	0.172	mg
Niacin	3.842	mg
Pyridoxine (Vitamin B6)	0.123	mg
Folate (Total)	74.343	µg
Cobalamin (Vitamin B12)	0.050	µg
Biotin	4.980	µg
Pantothenic Acid	1.007	mg
Vitamin K	109.658	µg
Phosphorus	98.260	mg
Magnesium	30.743	mg
Zinc	0.695	mg
Copper	0.144	mg
Manganese	0.257	mg
Selenium	2.587	µg
Chromium	0.001	mg

Combine all dressing ingredients, mixing until uniform. Divide the arugula among 4 bowls. Arrange the salad with arugula at the bottom, then layering the mushrooms, sprouts, and feta cheese. Top each serving with 2 tablespoons of dressing. Refrigerate any leftover dressing for later use.

Serves 4.

Recipe Tidbit:

You can find enoki mushrooms at an Asian market or at some gourmet groceries. If this isn't possible, just use nice-looking crimini mushrooms.

CUCUMBER JICAMA FRUIT SALAD

INGREDIENTS

2 cups peeled, cubed jicama

2 English cucumbers, cut into slices

2 cups blueberries

2 cups strawberries, center whites removed, cut into small chunks

2 teaspoons fresh lime juice

Place all ingredients except lime juice in a bowl, and mix very lightly to combine. Sprinkle with lime juice, and serve immediately.

Serves 4.

Recipe Tidbit:

This recipe works best if all ingredients are cold, so make sure your ingredients are in the refrigerator for at least an hour before preparing. Avoid overstirring to prevent the strawberries from getting mushy. You can make this salad ahead of time, but it is truly best if eaten very fresh.

Macronutrients		
Kilocalories	112.159	kcal
Trans Fatty Acid		g
Sugar, Total		g
Protein	2.474	g
Carbohydrate	27.419	g
Fat, Total	0.681	g
Alcohol	0.000	g
Cholesterol	0.000	mg
Saturated Fat	0.101	g
Monounsaturated Fat	0.076	g
Polyunsaturated Fat	0.294	g
Dietary Fiber, Total	7.112	g
Sugar, Total	14.463	g

Percentage of Kcals	
Protein	7.9%
Carbohydrate	87.3%
Fat, total	4.9%
Alcohol	0.0%

Vitamins & Minerals		
Sodium	7.093	mg
Potassium	487.238	mg
Vitamin A (RE)	22.068	RE
Vitamin C	67.417	mg
Calcium	48.071	mg
Iron	1.310	mg
Vitamin D (ug)	0.000	µg
Thiamin	0.098	mg
Riboflavin	0.114	mg
Niacin	0.861	mg
Pyridoxine (Vitamin B6)	0.160	mg
Folate (Total)	40.183	µg
Cobalamin (Vitamin B12)	0.000	µg
Biotin	0.793	µg
Pantothenic Acid	0.660	mg
Vitamin K	40.468	µg
Phosphorus	74.101	mg
Magnesium	41.242	mg
Zinc	0.623	mg
Copper	0.169	mg
Manganese	0.680	mg
Selenium	1.267	µg
Molybdenum	9.665	µg

CUCUMBER AVOCADO SALAD

INGREDIENTS

1 large avocado or 2 small, cubed

1 large cucumber, chopped

1 tomato, chopped (optional)

1 clove garlic, minced

½ cup minced cilantro, stems removed

½ teaspoon fresh lime juice

salt and pepper to taste

When selecting the avocado for this salad, I try to pick one that is barely ripe—not overripe—so that when I cube it, it doesn't get mushy. Stir together avocado, cucumber, garlic, and tomato (if you are using it). Lightly toss with cilantro and lime juice, and season with salt and pepper.

Macronutrients		
Kilocalories	74.373	kcal
Trans Fatty Acid		g
Sugar, Total		g
Protein	1.508	g
Carbohydrate	7.191	g
Fat, Total	5.309	g
Alcohol	0.000	g
Cholesterol	0.000	mg
Saturated Fat	0.748	g
Monounsaturated Fat	3.288	g
Polyunsaturated Fat	0.659	g
Dietary Fiber, Total	3.092	g
Sugar, Total	2.184	g

Percentage of Kcals	
Protein	7.3%
Carbohydrate	34.8%
Fat, total	57.9%
Alcohol	0.0%

Vitamins & Minerals		
Sodium	5.856	mg
Potassium	356.695	mg
Vitamin A (RE)	38.467	RE
Vitamin C	9.687	mg
Calcium	20.907	mg
Iron	0.511	mg
Vitamin D (ug)	0.000	µg
Thiamin	0.058	mg
Riboflavin	0.079	mg
Niacin	0.902	mg
Pyridoxine (Vitamin B6)	0.160	mg
Folate (Total)	39.711	µg
Cobalamin (Vitamin B12)	0.000	µg
Biotin	1.225	µg
Pantothenic Acid	0.716	mg
Vitamin K	21.805	µg
Phosphorus	44.724	mg
Magnesium	23.096	mg
Zinc	0.439	mg
Copper	0.108	mg
Manganese	0.157	mg
Selenium	0.467	µg
Chromium	0.007	mg

Serves 4.

Recipe Tidbit:

If you are following an anti-inflammatory diet, simply omit the tomato.

Chapter 4

SOUPS

SIMPLE VEGETABLE BROTH

INGREDIENTS

1 pound green beans

2 pounds zucchini, diced large

3 stalks celery, diced large

1 onion, diced large

1 bunch parsley

4 cloves garlic, diced large

1 teaspoon grated ginger

4 cups filtered water

2 tablespoons coconut oil or
organic butter

Macronutrients		
Kilocalories	68.601	kcal
Trans Fatty Acid		g
Sugar, Total		g
Protein	0.598	g
Carbohydrate	2.046	g
Fat, Total	6.919	g
Alcohol	0.000	g
Cholesterol	0.000	mg
Saturated Fat	5.912	g
Monounsaturated Fat	0.404	g
Polyunsaturated Fat	0.161	g
Trans Fatty Acid	0.000	g
Dietary Fiber, Total	0.685	g
Sugar, Total	1.110	g
Percentage of Kcals		
Protein	3.3%	
Carbohydrate	11.2%	
Fat, total	85.5%	
Alcohol	0.0%	
Vitamins & Minerals		
Sodium	13.023	mg
Potassium	107.137	mg
Vitamin A (RE)	26.520	RE
Vitamin C	7.857	mg
Calcium	19.416	mg
Iron	0.315	mg
Vitamin D (ug)	0.000	µg
Thiamin	0.023	mg
Riboflavin	0.037	mg
Niacin	0.221	mg
Pyridoxine (Vitamin B6)	0.064	mg
Folate (Total)	13.113	µg
Cobalamin (Vitamin B12)	0.000	µg
Biotin	0.034	µg
Pantothenic Acid	0.091	mg
Vitamin K	28.465	µg
Phosphorus	15.802	mg
Magnesium	10.749	mg
Zinc	0.128	mg
Copper	0.046	mg
Manganese	0.079	mg
Selenium	0.184	µg
Chromium	0.001	mg
Molybdenum	0.050	µg

Combine all vegetables with water in a large soup pot; bring to a boil over medium-high heat. Reduce heat and simmer for at least 30 minutes or until vegetables are soft. Using a colander, strain broth from vegetables and discard vegetables. Add the butter or coconut oil. Use immediately, or freeze in small batches for future use. If you want thicker broth, keep about a quarter of the vegetables, and puree into the broth using a high-powered blender or an immersion (handheld) blender.

Serves 4.

SAUSAGE SOUP

INGREDIENTS

4 tablespoons unsalted butter

1 red onion, minced

6 cloves garlic, minced

3 shallots, minced

4 large carrots, diced

4 stalks celery, diced

1 pound bulk chicken or turkey
  sausage

1 teaspoon thyme

1 teaspoon oregano

1 teaspoon basil

1 teaspoon celery seed

6 cups filtered water

3 cups kale, chopped

1 15-ounce can Navy beans

1 15-ounce can diced tomatoes

Macronutrients		
Kilocalories	261.189	kcal
Trans Fatty Acid		g
Sugar, Total		g
Protein	17.849	g
Carbohydrate	21.897	g
Fat, Total	12.120	g
Alcohol	0.000	g
Cholesterol	63.864	mg
Saturated Fat	5.395	g
Monounsaturated Fat	1.583	g
Polyunsaturated Fat	0.476	g
Trans Fatty Acid	0.233	g
Dietary Fiber, Total	5.885	g
Sugar, Total	4.670	g
Percentage of Kcals		
Protein	26.6%	
Carbohydrate	32.7%	
Fat, total	40.7%	
Alcohol	0.0%	
Vitamins & Minerals		
Sodium	692.957	mg
Potassium	483.517	mg
Vitamin A (RE)	858.430	RE
Vitamin C	39.051	mg
Calcium	129.205	mg
Iron	3.066	mg
Vitamin D (ug)	0.107	µg
Thiamin	0.143	mg
Riboflavin	0.105	mg
Niacin	0.951	mg
Pyridoxine (Vitamin B6)	0.245	mg
Folate (Total)	87.126	µg
Cobalamin (Vitamin B12)	0.012	µg
Biotin	0.935	µg
Pantothenic Acid	0.282	mg
Vitamin K	196.528	µg
Phosphorus	123.734	mg
Magnesium	50.633	mg
Zinc	0.767	mg
Copper	0.550	mg
Manganese	0.539	mg
Selenium	3.977	µg
Chromium	0.008	mg
Molybdenum	2.968	µg

Sweat the onion, garlic, and shallots in the butter over medium-low heat. Add the carrots, celery, sausage, and herbs, and continue to cook while teasing apart any large chunks of sausage. Once sausage is cooked through and beginning to brown, add water and simmer for 5 minutes to allow flavors to mingle. Add kale, beans, and tomatoes, and heat another 3 minutes. Serve warm.

Serves 8.

Recipe Tidbit:
  I included a lot of butter in this recipe because it adds flavor and fat, which help to curb sugar cravings.

CHICKEN NO-NODDLE SOUP

INGREDIENTS

½ onion, minced

4 garlic cloves, minced

2 tablespoons butter

3 large carrots, diced

3 large stalks celery, diced

1 teaspoon celery seed

1 teaspoon thyme

4 14-ounce cans organic
chicken broth

2 cups cubed cooked chicken

fresh parsley, minced

Sweat the onion and garlic in butter over medium-low heat. Add the carrots, celery, and herbs, and sauté for another 5 minutes. Add the chicken broth and chicken, and simmer for 5 more minutes. Ladle into bowls, and top with fresh parsley before serving.

Serves 4.

Recipe Tidbit:

You can add many different types of vegetables to this soup. Greens such as kale or chard are a great addition. I like a high ratio of vegetables to broth, so my soups are usually pretty hearty.

Macronutrients		
Kilocalories	236.595	kcal
Trans Fatty Acid		g
Sugar, Total		g
Protein	23.638	g
Carbohydrate	9.674	g
Fat, Total	10.798	g
Alcohol	0.000	g
Cholesterol	73.365	mg
Saturated Fat	4.994	g
Monounsaturated Fat	3.265	g
Polyunsaturated Fat	1.404	g
Trans Fatty Acid	0.233	g
Dietary Fiber, Total	2.246	g
Sugar, Total	4.886	g

Percentage of Kcals	
Protein	41.0%
Carbohydrate	16.8%
Fat, total	42.2%
Alcohol	0.0%

Vitamins & Minerals		
Sodium	1114.950	mg
Potassium	900.731	mg
Vitamin A (RE)	842.915	RE
Vitamin C	5.843	mg
Calcium	62.644	mg
Iron	2.363	mg
Vitamin D (ug)	0.177	µg
Vitamin E (mg)	0.165	mg
Thiamin	0.087	mg
Riboflavin	0.170	mg
Niacin	4.900	mg
Pyridoxine (Vitamin B6)	0.327	mg
Folate (Total)	27.617	µg
Cobalamin (Vitamin B12)	0.166	µg
Biotin	1.555	µg
Pantothenic Acid	0.764	mg
Vitamin K	23.113	µg
Phosphorus	141.933	mg
Magnesium	28.727	mg
Zinc	1.663	mg
Copper	0.098	mg
Manganese	0.243	mg
Selenium	15.438	µg
Chromium	0.013	mg
Molybdenum	4.452	µg

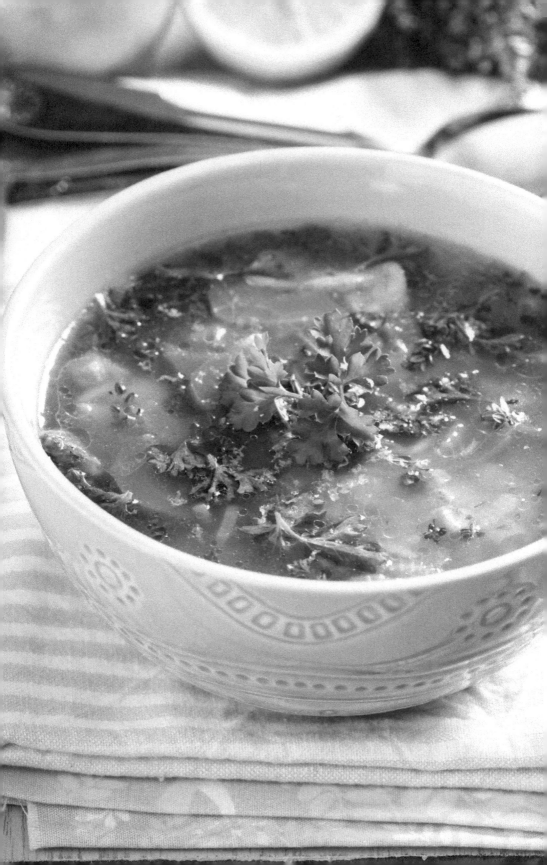

THAI RED CURRY SOUP

INGREDIENTS

1 13.5-ounce can full-fat coconut milk

2 tablespoons Thai red curry paste

3 cups organic chicken broth

1 onion, chopped

4 Kaffir lime leaves (find at a Thai or Asian market)

6 ounces raw pumpkin, chopped

5 ounces green beans, chopped

1 red bell pepper, cut into strips

3 small zucchinis, chopped

1 cup bok choy, chopped

2 tablespoons fresh basil leaves, whole or cut in halves

1 tablespoon fresh lemon juice

½ teaspoon fish sauce (no sugar added)

½ teaspoon salt

stevia (optional)

Macronutrients		
Kilocalories	156.266	kcal
Trans Fatty Acid		g
Sugar, Total		g
Protein	4.599	g
Carbohydrate	11.520	g
Fat, Total	9.311	g
Alcohol	0.000	g
Cholesterol	0.000	mg
Saturated Fat	8.114	g
Monounsaturated Fat	0.021	g
Polyunsaturated Fat	0.149	g
Trans Fatty Acid	0.000	g
Dietary Fiber, Total	3.006	g
Sugar, Total	8.145	g

Percentage of Kcals	
Protein	12.4%
Carbohydrate	31.1%
Fat, total	56.5%
Alcohol	0.0%

Vitamins & Minerals		
Sodium	890.497	mg
Potassium	599.453	mg
Vitamin A (RE)	176.098	RE
Vitamin C	58.356	mg
Calcium	53.253	mg
Iron	1.854	mg
Vitamin D (ug)	0.000	µg
Vitamin E (mg)	0.301	mg
Thiamin	0.134	mg
Riboflavin	0.148	mg
Niacin	0.937	mg
Pyridoxine (Vitamin B6)	0.304	mg
Folate (Total)	56.580	µg
Cobalamin (Vitamin B12)	0.000	µg
Biotin	0.329	µg
Pantothenic Acid	0.470	mg
Vitamin K	28.565	µg
Phosphorus	67.478	mg
Magnesium	33.867	mg
Zinc	0.546	mg
Copper	0.092	mg
Manganese	0.329	mg
Selenium	0.514	µg
Chromium	0.008	mg

Combine coconut milk, curry paste, and chicken broth in a large wok or saucepan. Bring to a boil, stirring occasionally. Add onion and lime leaves, and boil for 3 more minutes. Add pumpkin, and simmer over medium heat for 8 minutes or until nearly cooked. Add beans, red bell pepper, and zucchini, and simmer for another 5 minutes. Add bok choy and basil and continue cooking until they are warmed. Add remaining ingredients, taste, and adjust seasonings as necessary.

Serves 6.

Recipe Tidbit:

You can make this soup without the Kaffir lime leaves, but they do add a distinctive flavor. You can also use different vegetables—whatever you have in your crisper drawer. To lessen the spiciness, reduce the amount of red curry paste.

Many brands of fish sauce contain sugar. Find a fish sauce online that doesn't. If you can't find one, substitute a teaspoon of anchovy paste and additional salt.

This soup is traditionally a little sweet. If you wish, you can add a small amount of stevia.

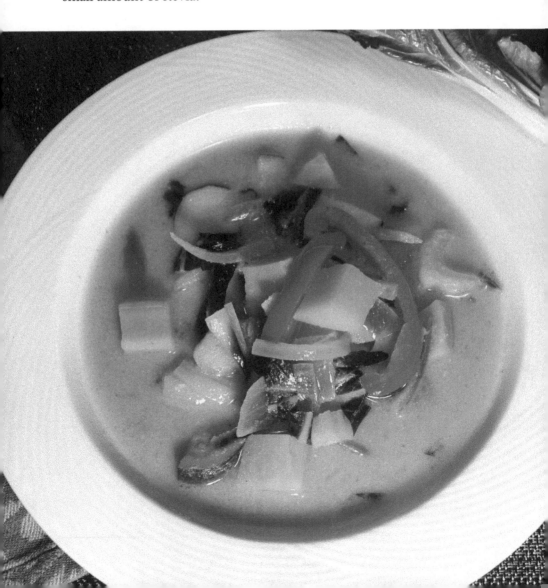

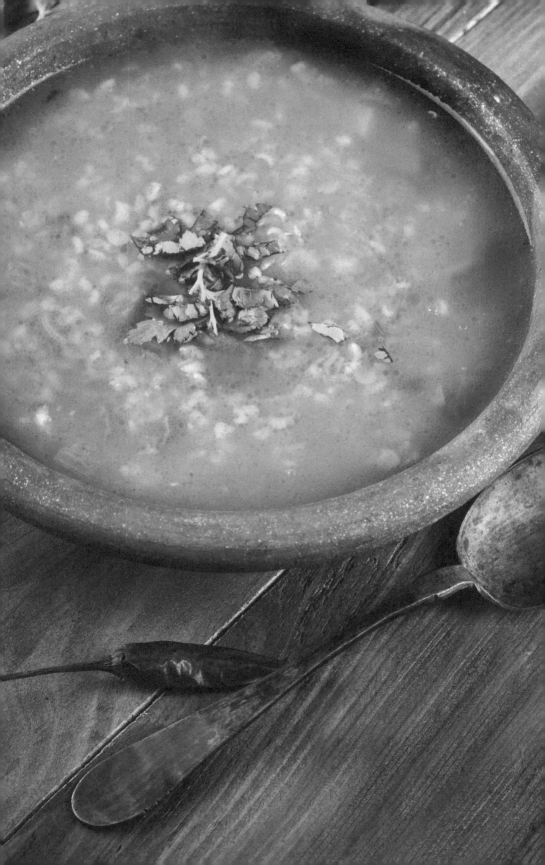

RED LENTIL SOUP

INGREDIENTS

3 tablespoons olive oil

1 red onion, chopped

2 cloves garlic, minced

1½ cups red lentils, sifted through your hands to remove small stones

1 tart peach, chopped

5 cups vegetable broth (recipe on page 106)

½ teaspoon ground cumin

½ teaspoon dried thyme

3 plum tomatoes, peeled, seeded, and chopped

2 tablespoons fresh lemon juice

salt and ground black pepper to taste

Macronutrients		
Kilocalories	329.124	kcal
Trans Fatty Acid		g
Sugar, Total		g
Protein	15.088	g
Carbohydrate	9.017	g
Fat, Total	13.516	g
Alcohol	0.000	g
Cholesterol	0.000	mg
Saturated Fat	6.007	g
Monounsaturated Fat	5.414	g
Polyunsaturated Fat	1.209	g
Trans Fatty Acid	0.000	g
Dietary Fiber, Total	2.142	g
Sugar, Total	6.918	g

Percentage of Kcals	
Protein	27.7%
Carbohydrate	16.5%
Fat, total	55.8%
Alcohol	0.0%

Vitamins & Minerals		
Sodium	35.893	mg
Potassium	725.762	mg
Vitamin A (RE)	87.812	RE
Vitamin C	20.317	mg
Calcium	63.017	mg
Iron	5.042	mg
Vitamin D (ug)	0.000	µg
Thiamin	0.344	mg
Riboflavin	0.171	mg
Niacin	1.923	mg
Pyridoxine (Vitamin B6)	0.486	mg
Folate (Total)	45.847	µg
Cobalamin (Vitamin B12)	0.000	µg
Biotin	2.978	µg
Pantothenic Acid	0.952	mg
Vitamin K	35.384	µg
Phosphorus	221.853	mg
Magnesium	67.677	mg
Zinc	2.064	mg
Copper	0.433	mg
Manganese	0.178	mg
Selenium	3.824	µg
Chromium	0.017	mg
Molybdenum	0.042	µg

Sweat onion and garlic in olive oil on medium-low heat for about 5 minutes. Add lentils, peach, and broth. Bring to a boil. Add cumin and thyme; reduce heat and simmer, covered, for 30 minutes, stirring occasionally. Add tomatoes and simmer 10 minutes more. Add lemon juice, salt, and pepper.

Pour half of the soup into a blender, and puree. Stir the pureed soup back into the rest of the soup, and serve warm.

Serves 6.

Recipe Tidbit:

The peach should be near ripe but not completely ripe or overripe. A peach that is still a little hard will be tarter.

BUTTERNUT SQUASH SOUP

INGREDIENTS

2 pounds butternut squash (about one large butternut squash)

1 red onion, minced

3 cloves garlic, minced

2 tablespoons butter

1½ cups chicken broth

⅓ cup half and half

1 tablespoon lemon juice

1 teaspoon salt

¼ teaspoon allspice

¼ teaspoon cardamom

Macronutrients		
Kilocalories	184.333	kcal
Trans Fatty Acid		g
Sugar, Total		g
Protein	3.791	g
Carbohydrate	27.260	g
Fat, Total	8.333	g
Alcohol	0.000	g
Cholesterol	22.719	mg
Saturated Fat	5.148	g
Monounsaturated Fat	2.181	g
Polyunsaturated Fat	0.396	g
Trans Fatty Acid	0.233	g
Dietary Fiber, Total	4.396	g
Sugar, Total	6.721	g

Percentage of Kcals	
Protein	7.6%
Carbohydrate	54.7%
Fat, total	37.6%
Alcohol	0.0%

Vitamins & Minerals		
Sodium	858.287	mg
Potassium	866.800	mg
Vitamin A (RE)	1998.413	RE
Vitamin C	38.471	mg
Calcium	126.537	mg
Iron	1.613	mg
Vitamin D (ug)	0.147	µg
Vitamin E (mg)	0.165	mg
Thiamin	0.197	mg
Riboflavin	0.079	mg
Niacin	2.246	mg
Pyridoxine (Vitamin B6)	0.350	mg
Folate (Total)	50.637	µg
Cobalamin (Vitamin B12)	0.079	µg
Pantothenic Acid	0.846	mg
Vitamin K	3.003	µg
Phosphorus	95.783	mg
Magnesium	70.924	mg
Zinc	0.481	mg
Copper	0.159	mg
Manganese	0.462	mg
Selenium	1.877	µg

Preheat oven to 375ºF. Prepare butternut squash by slicing it in half and digging out the inner pulp. Place both halves face down in a baking pan filled with at least 1½ inches of water, and transfer to oven. Wet-roast the squash until tender, about 45 minutes. Remove from oven and allow to cool slightly before cutting into cubes.

Sweat onions and garlic in butter in a sauté pan over medium-low heat for about 5 minutes; remove from heat. Place prepared squash and all other ingredients in a high-powered blender, and blend until smooth. Taste, and adjust seasonings as desired.

Serves 4.

Recipe Tidbit:

Be careful when using a blender to puree hot ingredients; they may explode when the blender is turned on. (This won't happen with a Vitamix.) Allow squash to cool slightly before blending, and then reheat the soup for serving. Alternatively, puree hot ingredients in very small batches, filling the blender container no more than ¼ full per batch.

If you want to omit the dairy, full-fat coconut milk works very well.

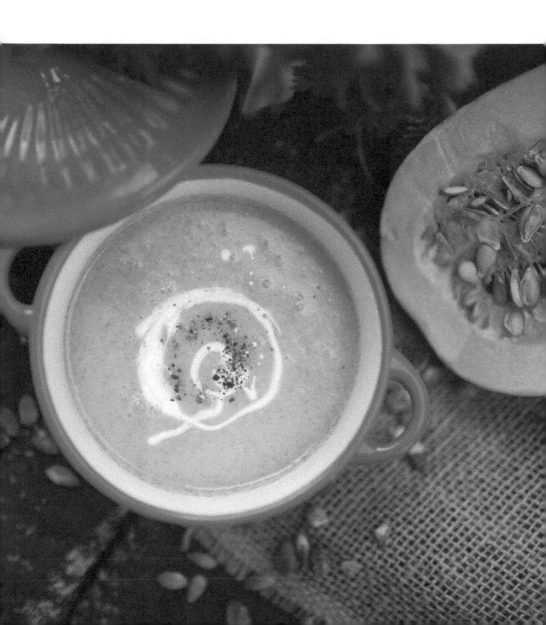

CHICKEN LENTIL SOUP

INGREDIENTS

4 tablespoons butter

1 large onion, diced

6 garlic cloves, thinly sliced

2 stalks celery, diced

2 carrots, diced

6 large chard leaves and stems, chopped, and stems separated from leaves

12 cups chicken stock or water

2 cups French green lentils, sifted through your hands to remove small stones

1 pound boneless, skinless chicken thighs, cut into 1-inch pieces

1 14-ounce can diced tomatoes

fresh parsley, minced

Macronutrients		
Kilocalories	445.961	kcal
Trans Fatty Acid		g
Sugar, Total		g
Protein	37.603	g
Carbohydrate	11.786	g
Fat, Total	12.390	g
Alcohol	0.000	g
Cholesterol	96.184	mg
Saturated Fat	5.864	g
Monounsaturated Fat	3.325	g
Polyunsaturated Fat	1.687	g
Trans Fatty Acid	0.328	g
Dietary Fiber, Total	2.941	g
Sugar, Total	5.936	g

Percentage of Kcals	
Protein	48.7%
Carbohydrate	15.3%
Fat, total	36.1%
Alcohol	0.0%

Vitamins & Minerals		
Sodium	384.211	mg
Potassium	1251.401	mg
Vitamin A (RE)	928.535	RE
Vitamin C	25.430	mg
Calcium	138.213	mg
Iron	10.556	mg
Vitamin D (ug)	0.142	µg
Vitamin E (mg)	0.220	mg
Thiamin	0.425	mg
Riboflavin	0.429	mg
Niacin	6.552	mg
Pyridoxine (Vitamin B6)	1.203	mg
Folate (Total)	109.159	µg
Cobalamin (Vitamin B12)	0.348	µg
Biotin	1.135	µg
Pantothenic Acid	1.243	mg
Vitamin K	409.914	µg
Phosphorus	445.086	mg
Magnesium	147.056	mg
Zinc	4.577	mg
Copper	0.948	mg
Manganese	1.408	mg
Selenium	99.479	µg
Chromium	0.012	mg
Molybdenum	2.539	µg

Sweat the onion in butter over medium heat for a few minutes. Add the garlic and sauté for a couple more minutes. Add the celery, carrots, and chard stems, and sauté for another 5 minutes. Add the chicken stock and lentils, and bring to a boil for at least 3 minutes. Reduce to a simmer, add chicken, chard greens, and diced tomatoes, and simmer on low until chicken and lentils are cooked, about 45 to 60 minutes. Ladle into bowls, and top with fresh parsley to serve.

Serves 6.

Recipe Tidbit:

I think garlic and lentils pair superbly; therefore, I use quite a bit of garlic in this recipe. You can use less if you wish. Experiment with using many different types of vegetables in this soup.

SPLIT PEA DAL WITH KALE

INGREDIENTS

Dal is the Hindi word for dried legumes. This variation on split pea soup is fragrant with traditional Indian spaces.

1 cup split peas, sifted through your hands to remove small stones

6 cups filtered water

1 teaspoon minced fresh ginger

1 teaspoon minced fresh jalapeño

1 teaspoon turmeric

1 teaspoon coriander

1½ teaspoon salt

2 tablespoons butter

½ teaspoon mustard seeds

½ teaspoon cumin seeds

4 cups loosely packed kale, stems removed and leaves chopped

1 13.5-ounce can full-fat coconut milk

1 teaspoon fresh lime juice

sour cream (optional)

Macronutrients		
Kilocalories	266.764	kcal
Trans Fatty Acid		g
Sugar, Total		g
Protein	10.445	g
Carbohydrate	26.252	g
Fat, Total	13.552	g
Alcohol	0.000	g
Cholesterol	10.177	mg
Saturated Fat	10.513	g
Monounsaturated Fat	1.186	g
Polyunsaturated Fat	0.489	g
Trans Fatty Acid	0.155	g
Dietary Fiber, Total	9.831	g
Sugar, Total	5.219	g

Percentage of Kcals	
Protein	15.5%
Carbohydrate	39.1%
Fat, total	45.4%
Alcohol	0.0%

Vitamins & Minerals		
Sodium	661.276	mg
Potassium	503.891	mg
Vitamin A (RE)	487.752	RE
Vitamin C	55.757	mg
Calcium	91.755	mg
Iron	3.148	mg
Vitamin D (ug)	0.071	µg
Vitamin E (mg)	0.110	mg
Thiamin	0.284	mg
Riboflavin	0.132	mg
Niacin	1.409	mg
Pyridoxine (Vitamin B6)	0.182	mg
Folate (Total)	150.720	µg
Cobalamin (Vitamin B12)	0.008	µg
Pantothenic Acid	0.609	mg
Vitamin K	321.269	µg
Phosphorus	148.688	mg
Magnesium	42.359	mg
Zinc	1.426	mg
Copper	0.959	mg
Manganese	0.774	mg
Selenium	2.384	µg

Wash the split peas thoroughly and drain. Combine with water in a large saucepan; cover and soak during the day so you are ready to make dinner when you come home from work.

Keep the split peas in the soaking water. Add ginger, jalapeño, turmeric, coriander, and salt, and bring to a boil over medium to high heat. Reduce heat and simmer until the peas are soft, about 40 to 50 minutes. While the dal is cooking, in a separate pan sauté the mustard seeds and cumin seeds in butter over medium heat for 4 to 7 minutes, stirring often to prevent the seeds from burning. I use a lid to make sure the seeds don't pop out of the pan. Add the kale leaves, coconut milk, lime juice, and butter-seed mixture to the dal; stir, cover, and remove from heat. Allow to sit for at least 5 minutes to soften the kale. Spoon into bowls, and top each serving with a dollop of sour cream if desired.

Recipe Tidbit:

People who regularly eat legumes may have a lower risk for diabetes. Split green peas have a low glycemic index, which means they do not cause rapid spikes in blood sugar. (I discuss glycemic index in depth in the book *The Freedom Diet*.) Split peas also contain 16.1 grams of dietary fiber per serving. Fiber both supports gastrointestinal health and helps to slow down sugar absorption, warding off those spikes in blood glucose.

Chapter 5:
ENTREES

CHICKEN LETTUCE WRAPS

INGREDIENTS

1 tablespoon butter

3 cloves garlic, minced

2 shallots, minced

2 stalks celery, diced

1 pound boneless, skinless chicken
   breast, cut into ½-inch pieces

½ teaspoon gluten-free tamari
   (soy sauce)

1 head butter lettuce

fresh cilantro, stems removed, chopped

For the sauce:

1 garlic clove, minced

2 tablespoons gluten-free tamari

1 tablespoon rice vinegar

1 tablespoon lemon juice

1 teaspoon sesame seeds

½ teaspoon grated fresh ginger

½ teaspoon red chili paste (available in
   the Asian section of most groceries)

⅛ teaspoon toasted sesame oil

Macronutrients		
Kilocalories	251.115	kcal
Trans Fatty Acid		g
Sugar, Total		g
Protein	37.055	g
Carbohydrate	5.479	g
Fat, Total	8.418	g
Alcohol	0.000	g
Cholesterol	120.306	mg
Saturated Fat	3.331	g
Monounsaturated Fat	2.190	g
Polyunsaturated Fat	1.122	g
Trans Fatty Acid	0.166	g
Dietary Fiber, Total	1.480	g
Sugar, Total	1.572	g
Percentage of Kcals		
Protein	60.3%	
Carbohydrate	8.9%	
Fat, total	30.8%	
Alcohol	0.0%	
Vitamins & Minerals		
Sodium	796.152	mg
Potassium	653.356	mg
Vitamin A (RE)	241.328	RE
Vitamin C	8.102	mg
Calcium	57.816	mg
Iron	2.051	mg
Vitamin D (ug)	0.071	µg
Vitamin E (mg)	0.349	mg
Thiamin	0.158	mg
Riboflavin	0.300	mg
Niacin	11.986	mg
Pyridoxine (Vitamin B6)	1.128	mg
Folate (Total)	61.979	µg
Cobalamin (Vitamin B12)	0.214	µg
Biotin	1.657	µg
Pantothenic Acid	2.464	mg
Vitamin K	64.177	µg
Phosphorus	300.016	mg
Magnesium	48.199	mg
Zinc	1.330	mg
Copper	0.131	mg
Manganese	0.254	mg
Selenium	35.950	µg
Chromium	0.017	mg
Molybdenum	1.430	µg

Combine ingredients for sauce, and set aside. Sweat the garlic and shallots in butter over medium-low heat for 5 minutes. Add the celery and sauté for another 3 minutes. Add the chicken and tamari, and continue sautéing until the chicken is cooked through, about 7 to 9 minutes. Spoon the chicken mixture into the lettuce leaves, and top each serving with 1 tablespoon of sauce and chopped cilantro leaves.

Serves 3.

ROMAINE SANDWICH

INGREDIENTS

1 romaine heart, leaves separated
   into long "boats"
2 tablespoons mayonnaise
1 tablespoon mustard
⅔ pound nitrite-free deli
   lunchmeat
1 green bell pepper, seeds
   removed, sliced long

Spread mustard and mayonnaise onto romaine leaves. Top with lunchmeat and pepper slices, and curl romaine around ingredients. Enjoy immediately.

Serves 2.

Recipe Tidbit:
   Make these "sandwich wraps" in the morning for a great light lunch.
   Get creative by varying the ingredients.

Macronutrients		
Kilocalories	273.338	kcal
Trans Fatty Acid		g
Sugar, Total		g
Protein	22.609	g
Carbohydrate	14.279	g
Fat, Total	13.400	g
Alcohol	0.000	g
Cholesterol	59.822	mg
Saturated Fat	1.668	g
Monounsaturated Fat	2.493	g
Polyunsaturated Fat	6.272	g
Trans Fatty Acid	0.026	g
Dietary Fiber, Total	1.438	g
Sugar, Total	1.647	g

Percentage of Kcals	
Protein	33.7%
Carbohydrate	21.3%
Fat, total	45.0%
Alcohol	0.0%

Vitamins & Minerals		
Sodium	1253.216	mg
Potassium	133.105	mg
Vitamin A (RE)	76.602	RE
Vitamin C	48.101	mg
Calcium	13.759	mg
Iron	0.410	mg
Vitamin D (ug)	0.028	µg
Thiamin	0.053	mg
Riboflavin	0.029	mg
Niacin	0.347	mg
Pyridoxine (Vitamin B6)	0.144	mg
Folate (Total)	15.325	µg
Cobalamin (Vitamin B12)	0.017	µg
Biotin	1.840	µg
Pantothenic Acid	0.110	mg
Vitamin K	33.152	µg
Phosphorus	24.698	mg
Magnesium	10.528	mg
Zinc	0.160	mg
Copper	0.050	mg
Manganese	0.115	mg
Selenium	2.854	µg
Chromium	0.012	mg
Molybdenum	0.107	µg

ZUCCHINI LASAGNA

INGREDIENTS

¼ cup olive oil

1 red onion, chopped

1 cup mushrooms, chopped

5 cloves garlic, minced

1 pound chicken Italian sausage

½ head cauliflower, chopped small

¼ cup dry white wine or water

1 teaspoon dried basil

1 teaspoon dried oregano

1 16-ounce jar spaghetti sauce
(sugar free)

1 14.5-ounce can diced tomatoes,
undrained

2 large or 4 small zucchinis, sliced
thinly lengthwise to make lasagna
"noodles"

1 cup Parmesan or Romano cheese
(optional)

Macronutrients		
Kilocalories	182.323	kcal
Trans Fatty Acid		g
Sugar, Total		g
Protein	9.270	g
Carbohydrate	13.113	g
Fat, Total	10.171	g
Alcohol	0.506	g
Cholesterol	29.777	mg
Saturated Fat	1.878	g
Monounsaturated Fat	4.693	g
Polyunsaturated Fat	1.103	g
Trans Fatty Acid	0.000	g
Dietary Fiber, Total	2.139	g
Sugar, Total	3.835	g
Percentage of Kcals		
Protein	20.1%	
Carbohydrate	28.4%	
Fat, total	49.6%	
Alcohol	1.9%	
Vitamins & Minerals		
Sodium	367.952	mg
Potassium	275.011	mg
Vitamin A (RE)	45.926	RE
Vitamin C	22.570	mg
Calcium	37.991	mg
Iron	1.400	mg
Vitamin D (ug)	0.016	µg
Thiamin	0.097	mg
Riboflavin	0.121	mg
Niacin	1.623	mg
Pyridoxine (Vitamin B6)	0.178	mg
Folate (Total)	41.655	µg
Cobalamin (Vitamin B12)	0.003	µg
Biotin	0.029	µg
Pantothenic Acid	0.358	mg
Vitamin K	14.917	µg
Phosphorus	53.220	mg
Magnesium	19.953	mg
Zinc	0.391	mg
Copper	0.097	mg
Manganese	0.144	mg
Selenium	6.483	µg
Chromium	0.003	mg

Preheat oven to 350°F. Sauté onion and mushrooms in oil in a large skillet over medium heat until tender, about 5 minutes; pour off any excessive liquid produced by cooking the mushrooms. Add garlic, sausage, and cauliflower. Sauté until sausage is cooked through and browned, about 10 minutes. Add wine or water and herbs, and simmer until excess liquid is evaporated, about 3 minutes.

Combine spaghetti sauce and diced tomatoes in a medium bowl; add the sausage mixture. Spoon a small amount of sauce into a 13 x 9–inch pan. Top with a layer of zucchini. Top with another thin layer of sauce. Continue layering zucchini and sauce, saving ⅓ of the sauce for the top. Sprinkle with cheese, if desired. Bake 20–30 minutes or until sauce is bubbling and cheese is melted and just beginning to brown.

Serves 12.

Recipe Tidbit:

To make the "zucchini noodles," use either a knife or a vegetable peeler.

This simple, throw-together meal can tolerate lots of variations. I am a fan of how the cauliflower and mushrooms complement each other, but you can experiment with other vegetables. The sausage adds flavor but is not needed if you are concerned about the seasonings in the sausage or if you are vegetarian.

If you can't find sugar-free spaghetti sauce, use a 26-ounce can of diced tomatoes (in addition to the 13.5-ounce can) and season with more oregano, basil, garlic powder, onion powder, and salt. If you cannot tolerate tomatoes, you can easily substitute an organic puréed soup—for example, a roasted–red pepper soup.

TURMERIC LENTILS WITH CHARD

INGREDIENTS

2 cups red lentils, sifted through
your hands to remove small stones

4 cups vegetable broth (see recipe
on page 106)

2 tablespoons olive oil

1 tablespoon butter

1 tablespoon mustard seeds

1 onion, chopped

2 cloves garlic, minced

2 teaspoons turmeric

1 teaspoon ground coriander

½ teaspoon cumin

1 bunch Swiss chard, chopped

1 pound Italian chicken sausage,
cooked (optional)

salt to taste

Macronutrients		
Kilocalories	547.619	kcal
Trans Fatty Acid		g
Sugar, Total		g
Protein	29.066	g
Carbohydrate	7.173	g
Fat, Total	19.072	g
Alcohol	0.000	g
Cholesterol	7.633	mg
Saturated Fat	8.980	g
Monounsaturated Fat	6.876	g
Polyunsaturated Fat	1.822	g
Trans Fatty Acid	0.117	g
Dietary Fiber, Total	2.043	g
Sugar, Total	5.361	g
Percentage of Kcals		
Protein	36.7%	
Carbohydrate	9.1%	
Fat, total	54.2%	
Alcohol	0.0%	
Vitamins & Minerals		
Sodium	105.259	mg
Potassium	1058.122	mg
Vitamin A (RE)	139.161	RE
Vitamin C	14.994	mg
Calcium	106.129	mg
Iron	10.167	mg
Vitamin D (ug)	0.053	µg
Vitamin E (mg)	0.083	mg
Thiamin	0.633	mg
Riboflavin	0.296	mg
Niacin	2.729	mg
Pyridoxine (Vitamin B6)	0.819	mg
Folate (Total)	64.499	µg
Cobalamin (Vitamin B12)	0.006	µg
Biotin	0.340	µg
Pantothenic Acid	1.726	mg
Vitamin K	134.833	µg
Phosphorus	419.822	mg
Magnesium	130.272	mg
Zinc	3.961	mg
Copper	0.774	mg
Manganese	0.471	mg
Selenium	12.744	µg
Chromium	0.007	mg
Molybdenum	0.050	µg

Combine lentils and broth in a medium saucepan; heat to boiling. Reduce heat and simmer, covered, until liquid is absorbed, about 30 minutes.

Heat oil and butter in a large saucepan over medium-low heat until hot but not smoking; add mustard seeds, cover, and cook for about 1 minute. Add onion, garlic, and spices, and sauté until onion is tender, about 5 minutes. Stir in chard and sausage (if using). Cook, stirring occasionally, until chard is wilted, about 2 minutes. Add lentils and cook about 5 minutes, until flavors are mingled. Season to taste with salt.

Serves 4.

Recipe Tidbit:

This is one of my favorite meals to make when I haven't gone grocery shopping. I'm partial to lentils. They don't have to be soaked, so they are easy to prepare quickly and are especially delicious when cooked in a flavored broth. Lentils are high in iron, amino acids, and B vitamins. They help to stabilize blood sugar and have been shown to improve cholesterol levels. I always keep them on hand. I usually also have some form of greens suitable for cooking.

I have experimented with this recipe in various ways, and they all turn out well. It's easy to make this dish vegetarian by eliminating the sausage. Play around with using different spices, different types of greens, and different types of lentils. You can dilute the broth to half strength with water, which will help the liquid absorb into the lentils more easily.

GREEN CURRY

I have made this curry many times. Its long list of ingredients may seem daunting, but it is actually very quick and easy to prepare and very versatile; you can change the veggies and protein source each time you make it. If you are worried about its being too spicy for kids, omit the jalapeño from the paste and add it instead to the hot sauce, which is served on the side.

INGREDIENTS

2 tablespoons coconut oil

Green Curry Paste (recipe follows)

1 pound boneless, skinless chicken breast, sliced into ½-inch-thick strips

¾ 14-ounce can coconut milk

1 yellow bell pepper, julienned

3 small zucchinis, julienned

2 cups chopped broccoli florets

1 pint cherry tomatoes, halved

½ cup chicken broth (optional)

fish sauce and fresh lime juice, to taste (optional)

Hot Sauce (optional; recipe follows)

Green Curry Paste:
1 stalk lemongrass
½ cup chopped cilantro
½ cup chopped fresh basil
¼ cup chopped purple onion

Macronutrients		
Kilocalories	481.656	kcal
Trans Fatty Acid		g
Sugar, Total		g
Protein	33.326	g
Carbohydrate	17.889	g
Fat, Total	32.023	g
Alcohol	0.000	g
Cholesterol	82.597	mg
Saturated Fat	25.413	g
Monounsaturated Fat	2.103	g
Polyunsaturated Fat	1.202	g
Trans Fatty Acid	0.008	g
Dietary Fiber, Total	3.592	g
Sugar, Total	8.921	g

Percentage of Kcals	
Protein	27.0%
Carbohydrate	14.5%
Fat, total	58.5%
Alcohol	0.0%

Vitamins & Minerals		
Sodium	1163.147	mg
Potassium	1519.376	mg
Vitamin A (RE)	173.348	RE
Vitamin C	185.680	mg
Calcium	119.064	mg
Iron	6.020	mg
Vitamin D (ug)	0.000	µg
Vitamin E (mg)	1.048	mg
Thiamin	0.280	mg
Riboflavin	0.444	mg
Niacin	12.093	mg
Pyridoxine (Vitamin B6)	1.400	mg
Folate (Total)	123.322	µg
Cobalamin (Vitamin B12)	0.220	µg
Biotin	1.276	µg
Pantothenic Acid	2.763	mg
Vitamin K	76.239	µg
Phosphorus	450.188	mg
Magnesium	150.907	mg
Zinc	2.408	mg
Copper	0.517	mg
Manganese	1.497	mg
Selenium	29.254	µg
Chromium	0.012	mg

1 2-inch piece galangal root, sliced

5 cloves garlic

½ jalapeño pepper, seeded

½ teaspoon ground coriander

½ teaspoon ground cumin

½ teaspoon ground white pepper

3 tablespoons fish sauce

1 teaspoon anchovy paste (or 2 anchovy filets)

2 tablespoons lime juice

¼ 14-ounce can whole coconut milk

Hot Sauce:

3 tablespoons Green Curry Paste

1 jalapeño pepper, seeded

1 2-inch piece ginger root, peeled and sliced

¼ cup chopped red onion

2 cloves garlic

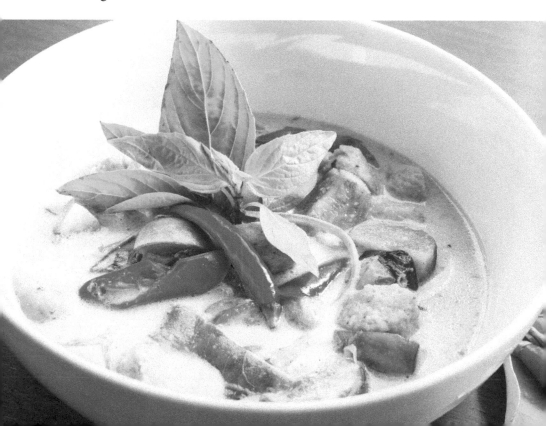

To make the curry paste, remove tough outer leaves from lemongrass and cut off the end. Finely chop the stalk. Combine lemongrass and remaining ingredients in a food processor or blender. Process until smooth, adding additional coconut milk as needed just to blend. To make the hot sauce, combine ingredients in a food processor or blender; process until smooth, adding a small amount of water if needed to blend. I usually make the green curry paste, remove it from the blender and leave just enough behind (3 tablespoons) to make the hot sauce.

Heat coconut oil in a wok or large skillet over medium-high heat until hot; stir in curry paste. (If you haven't already, reserve 3 table-spoons of paste for making the hot sauce.) Stir-fry until fragrant, 1–2 minutes. Add chicken and coconut milk; heat to boiling. Reduce heat and simmer 5 minutes. Add vegetables and simmer until chicken is cooked and vegetables are tender but remain crunchy, about 10 min-utes. If more liquid is needed or you want more sauce, add chicken broth, a couple of tablespoons at a time. Adjust flavors by adding fish sauce and/or lime juice to taste. Serve with hot sauce on the side.

Serves 4.

Recipe Tidbit:

Omit cherry tomatoes for individuals with arthritis or who are sensitive to tomatoes.

Most fish sauces are gluten-free; however, make sure to check the label for thickeners and sugar, and buy one without sugar.

Experiment with other vegetables—green beans, bamboo shoots, yellow squash, carrots, cabbage.

Galangal root can be found at an Asian market. I usually buy a few large roots, cut them into 2-inch pieces, and freeze them until I need them. I almost always double the curry paste recipe and freeze half for a future dinner.

HERBED BEEF

INGREDIENTS

2 tablespoons olive oil

½ onion, minced

1 pound organic grass-fed ground beef

3 garlic cloves, minced

½ teaspoon salt

½ teaspoon pepper

1 bunch parsley, stems removed, minced

3 cups kale, stems removed, leaves
  chopped

Sweat onion in olive oil for 3 minutes over medium heat. Add beef and garlic, and sauté until meat is no longer pink. Season with salt and pepper, and add parsley. Cook for just a couple of minutes, until parsley is bright green. Divide kale between three bowls, and evenly divide the beef between the bowls. Serve warm.

Serves 3.

Macronutrients		
Kilocalories	394.713	kcal
Trans Fatty Acid		g
Sugar, Total		g
Protein	32.960	g
Carbohydrate	9.432	g
Fat, Total	26.301	g
Alcohol	0.000	g
Cholesterol	90.805	mg
Saturated Fat	8.057	g
Monounsaturated Fat	12.768	g
Polyunsaturated Fat	1.897	g
Trans Fatty Acid	1.135	g
Dietary Fiber, Total	3.210	g
Sugar, Total	2.410	g

Percentage of Kcals	
Protein	32.5%
Carbohydrate	9.3%
Fat, total	58.3%
Alcohol	0.0%

Vitamins & Minerals		
Sodium	523.022	mg
Potassium	865.687	mg
Vitamin A (RE)	754.861	RE
Vitamin C	96.170	mg
Calcium	144.155	mg
Iron	4.799	mg
Vitamin D (ug)	0.000	µg
Thiamin	0.142	mg
Riboflavin	0.339	mg
Niacin	7.406	mg
Pyridoxine (Vitamin B6)	0.519	mg
Folate (Total)	119.856	µg
Cobalamin (Vitamin B12)	2.234	µg
Biotin	0.204	µg
Pantothenic Acid	1.018	mg
Vitamin K	646.181	µg
Phosphorus	342.572	mg
Magnesium	68.476	mg
Zinc	7.434	mg
Copper	1.136	mg
Manganese	0.592	mg
Selenium	22.619	µg
Chromium	0.005	mg

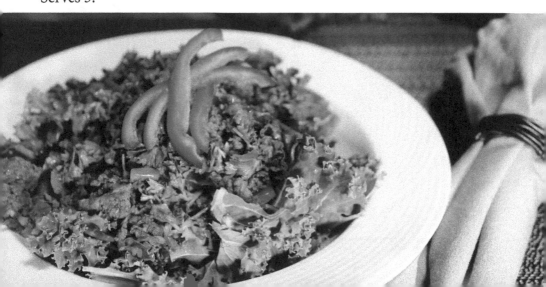

EASY CHILI

INGREDIENTS

1 tablespoon olive oil

2 small red onions, minced

4 cloves garlic, minced

2 large carrots, grated

2 zucchini, grated

2 pounds organic grass-fed ground
beef

2 26-ounce cartons diced tomatoes
or 2 28-ounce cans diced
tomatoes

2 packets chili seasoning (Simply
Organic Chili Seasoning, mild or
spicy)

2 packets ranch seasoning (Simply
Organic Ranch Seasoning)

2 15-ounce cans chili beans (1
15-ounce can pinto beans plus
1 15-ounce can kidney beans),
drained

Macronutrients		
Kilocalories	386.587	kcal
Trans Fatty Acid		g
Sugar, Total		g
Protein	28.865	g
Carbohydrate	34.417	g
Fat, Total	15.023	g
Alcohol	0.000	g
Cholesterol	68.104	mg
Saturated Fat	5.336	g
Monounsaturated Fat	5.841	g
Polyunsaturated Fat	0.771	g
Trans Fatty Acid	0.852	g
Dietary Fiber, Total	7.028	g
Sugar, Total	10.151	g

Percentage of Kcals	
Protein	29.7%
Carbohydrate	35.5%
Fat, total	34.8%
Alcohol	0.0%

Vitamins & Minerals		
Sodium	1631.606	mg
Potassium	557.396	mg
Vitamin A (RE)	509.827	RE
Vitamin C	27.145	mg
Calcium	149.134	mg
Iron	5.336	mg
Vitamin D (ug)	0.000	µg
Thiamin	0.083	mg
Riboflavin	0.245	mg
Niacin	5.394	mg
Pyridoxine (Vitamin B6)	0.354	mg
Folate (Total)	24.690	µg
Cobalamin (Vitamin B12)	1.675	µg
Biotin	0.458	µg
Pantothenic Acid	0.804	mg
Vitamin K	6.519	µg
Phosphorus	232.674	mg
Magnesium	35.321	mg
Zinc	5.417	mg
Copper	0.120	mg
Manganese	0.145	mg
Selenium	16.566	µg
Chromium	0.003	mg
Molybdenum	1.317	µg

Sauté onion and garlic in olive oil for 3 minutes over medium heat. Add carrots and zucchini, and sauté for another 5 minutes. Add ground beef, and sauté until beef has only a small amount of pink color remaining. Add tomatoes and seasonings, and simmer for at least 15 minutes, stirring occasionally. Add beans; stir, and simmer another 5 minutes. Serve warm over arugula, kale, collard greens, or another cooking green. Top with sour cream, fresh minced onions, or grated cheese, if desired.

Serves 8.

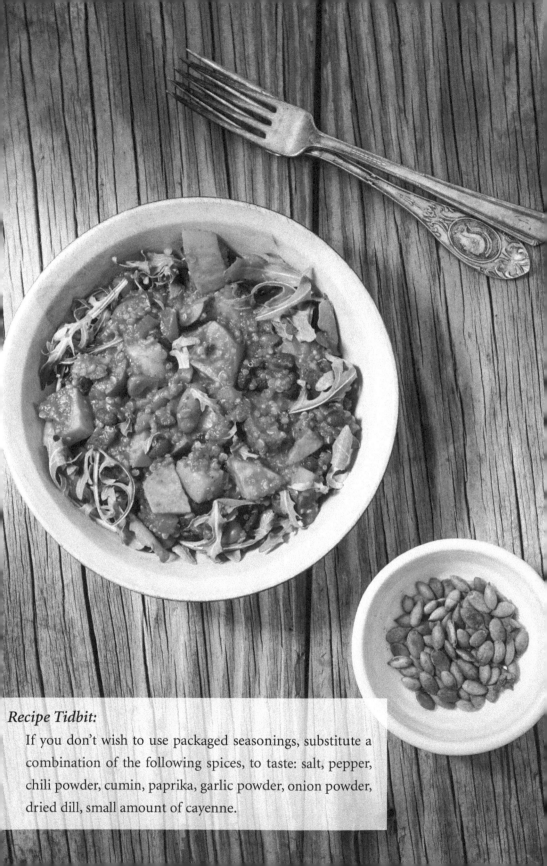

BAKED SALMON WITH BROCCOLI AND ARUGULA

INGREDIENTS

1 pound salmon filets

2 crowns broccoli, chopped

2 cups arugula

salt and pepper to taste

Rub mixture:

1 teaspoon onion powder

1 teaspoon garlic powder

1 teaspoon dried dill

1 teaspoon salt

1 teaspoon pepper

Macronutrients

Kilocalories	341.159	kcal
Trans Fatty Acid		g
Sugar, Total		g
Protein	33.002	g
Carbohydrate	5.695	g
Fat, Total	20.412	g
Alcohol	0.000	g
Cholesterol	82.168	mg
Saturated Fat	4.616	g
Monounsaturated Fat	5.663	g
Polyunsaturated Fat	5.866	g
Trans Fatty Acid	0.000	g
Dietary Fiber, Total	1.935	g
Sugar, Total	1.203	g

Percentage of Kcals

Protein	39.0%
Carbohydrate	6.7%
Fat, total	54.3%
Alcohol	0.0%

Vitamins & Minerals

Sodium	886.474	mg
Potassium	795.576	mg
Vitamin A (RE)	85.569	RE
Vitamin C	52.251	mg
Calcium	71.550	mg
Iron	1.393	mg
Vitamin D (ug)	0.000	µg
Thiamin	0.364	mg
Riboflavin	0.309	mg
Niacin	13.500	mg
Pyridoxine (Vitamin B6)	1.039	mg
Folate (Total)	83.492	µg
Cobalamin (Vitamin B12)	3.907	µg
Pantothenic Acid	2.709	mg
Vitamin K	67.553	µg
Phosphorus	412.032	mg
Magnesium	61.887	mg
Zinc	0.891	mg
Copper	0.123	mg
Manganese	0.288	mg
Selenium	37.942	µg
Chromium	0.012	mg

Combine ingredients for the rub in a small bowl. Gently rub the mixture into the salmon filets, using your fingers to massage it into the meat. Wrap the salmon in plastic wrap, and refrigerate for at least 12 hours.

Preheat oven to 350ºF. Bake the salmon, skin side down and covered, for about 12 minutes. Uncover and bake for another 3–5 minutes or until salmon is tender on the inside but no longer raw-pink.

While the salmon is baking, prepare the broccoli, steaming it in an inch or two of water over medium to high heat until it is bright green but still crunchy, about 4–5 minutes. Remove from heat, and immediately combine with arugula to wilt the greens. Season with salt and pepper as desired. Divide the vegetable mixture between three plates, and top with equal amounts of baked salmon. Serve with lemon wedges.

Serves 3.

EASY FRIED RICE

INGREDIENTS

2 eggs

⅛ teaspoon gluten-free tamari,
plus more to taste

⅛ teaspoon toasted sesame oil

3 tablespoons coconut oil, divided

¾ cup red onion, minced

2 celery stalks, minced

2 large carrots, minced

1 cup spinach, minced

1 cup frozen peas

3 cups cooked brown rice, cold

8 ounces cooked chicken breast,
cold, chopped

Macronutrients		
Kilocalories	430.239	kcal
Trans Fatty Acid		g
Sugar, Total		g
Protein	26.299	g
Carbohydrate	45.276	g
Fat, Total	16.019	g
Alcohol	0.000	g
Cholesterol	136.659	mg
Saturated Fat	10.423	g
Monounsaturated Fat	2.648	g
Polyunsaturated Fat	1.686	g
Trans Fatty Acid	0.010	g
Dietary Fiber, Total	6.538	g
Sugar, Total	5.124	g
Percentage of Kcals		
Protein	24.4%	
Carbohydrate	42.1%	
Fat, total	33.5%	
Alcohol	0.0%	
Vitamins & Minerals		
Sodium	161.374	mg
Potassium	470.347	mg
Vitamin A (RE)	716.577	RE
Vitamin C	10.082	mg
Calcium	76.045	mg
Iron	2.546	mg
Vitamin D (ug)	0.557	µg
Vitamin E (mg)	0.263	mg
Thiamin	0.327	mg
Riboflavin	0.307	mg
Niacin	8.090	mg
Pyridoxine (Vitamin B6)	0.584	mg
Folate (Total)	74.543	µg
Cobalamin (Vitamin B12)	0.353	µg
Biotin	1.451	µg
Pantothenic Acid	1.319	mg
Vitamin K	56.926	µg
Phosphorus	320.644	mg
Magnesium	102.237	mg
Zinc	2.237	mg
Copper	0.270	mg
Manganese	1.584	mg
Selenium	35.345	µg
Chromium	0.022	mg
Molybdenum	4.843	µg

Combine eggs with ⅛ teaspoon tamari and sesame oil, and beat just until combined. Heat 1 tablespoon of coconut oil in a wok or large skillet over medium heat. Add onions, and sweat until onions are translucent and begin to turn brown, about 5–8 minutes. Add celery and carrots, and sauté for another 5 minutes. Push vegetables to the sides of the pan; add 1 tablespoon of coconut oil and the egg mixture. Cook until the egg begins to get puffy; using a spatula, flip the egg. Cook for a bit longer on the other side, then cut into pieces in the pan and incorporate into vegetables. Add spinach and peas, and sauté for 1–2 minutes. Again push the vegetable-egg mixture to the sides, and add another tablespoon of coconut oil. Add rice and chicken, and cook without stirring for 3–5 minutes. Stir and cook for another 3–5 minutes, until chicken is warmed and rice has a lightly fried appearance. Add additional tamari to taste.

Serves 4.

Recipe Tidbit:

To make this recipe even healthier, serve it in lettuce wraps or over dark greens such as kale or chard.

JICAMA FISH TACOS

INGREDIENTS

1 large jicama, thinly sliced to
create round "taco chips" (see
instructions below)

1 pound fresh rainbow trout filets

1 tablespoon olive oil

pinch salt

pinch pepper

⅛ teaspoon thyme

2 teaspoons lemon juice

½ cup thinly sliced red cabbage

½ cup cilantro, stems removed,
minced

For the sauce:

½ cup minced cucumbers (remove
seeds before mincing)

½ cup fresh cilantro

¼ cup mayonnaise

1 tablespoon lime juice

2 teaspoons dried dill or 2 tablespoons fresh

1 clove garlic

½ teaspoon salt

½ teaspoon pepper

Macronutrients		
Kilocalories	474.390	kcal
Trans Fatty Acid		g
Sugar, Total		g
Protein	32.569	g
Carbohydrate	22.794	g
Fat, Total	27.847	g
Alcohol	0.000	g
Cholesterol	96.474	mg
Saturated Fat	4.913	g
Monounsaturated Fat	9.369	g
Polyunsaturated Fat	11.056	g
Trans Fatty Acid	0.105	g
Dietary Fiber, Total	11.497	g
Sugar, Total	4.981	g

Percentage of Kcals	
Protein	27.6%
Carbohydrate	19.3%
Fat, total	53.1%
Alcohol	0.0%

Vitamins & Minerals		
Sodium	595.693	mg
Potassium	997.790	mg
Vitamin A (RE)	140.665	RE
Vitamin C	58.761	mg
Calcium	91.215	mg
Iron	2.451	mg
Vitamin D (ug)	24.075	µg
Thiamin	0.238	mg
Riboflavin	0.222	mg
Niacin	8.965	mg
Pyridoxine (Vitamin B6)	0.642	mg
Folate (Total)	48.833	µg
Cobalamin (Vitamin B12)	6.198	µg
Biotin	2.447	µg
Pantothenic Acid	2.935	mg
Vitamin K	42.431	µg
Phosphorus	399.553	mg
Magnesium	73.068	mg
Zinc	1.168	mg
Copper	0.201	mg
Manganese	0.286	mg
Selenium	37.934	µg
Chromium	0.004	mg

To make the sauce, combine all ingredients except cucumber in a blender or food processor, and process until smooth. Stir in cucumber, and set aside.

Prepare jicama "chips" by slicing them thin. If you have a mandolin slicer this will be easier, but you can manage without. You may end up with leftover jicama, as the ends may be too small to make suitably sized chips. In this case, simply chop the remaining jicama, and serve on the side with salt and lime juice to taste.

Preheat oven to 400ºF. Line a baking pan with parchment paper. Rub olive oil on fish filet, and season with salt, pepper, thyme, and lemon juice. Add fish and a small amount of water to the baking pan, and bake in the oven for 7–12 minutes, until fish flakes easily with a fork. Remove from oven.

Prepare tacos by topping the jicama chips with fish, and then with cabbage and cilantro. Spoon sauce over each taco, and serve warm.

Serves 3.

SPAGHETTI SQUASH WITH MEAT SAUCE

INGREDIENTS

1 large or 2 small spaghetti squash

1 tablespoon olive oil

1 onion, minced

4 cloves garlic, minced

1 pound ground beef (organic and grass fed)

1 teaspoon basil

1 teaspoon oregano

1 teaspoon salt

1 26-ounce can diced tomatoes

4 cups chard, stems removed and chopped small

Macronutrients		
Kilocalories	304.200	kcal
Trans Fatty Acid		g
Sugar, Total		g
Protein	25.065	g
Carbohydrate	15.780	g
Fat, Total	16.167	g
Alcohol	0.000	g
Cholesterol	68.104	mg
Saturated Fat	5.596	g
Monounsaturated Fat	7.104	g
Polyunsaturated Fat	1.019	g
Trans Fatty Acid	0.852	g
Dietary Fiber, Total	3.379	g
Sugar, Total	6.185	g

Percentage of Kcals	
Protein	32.5%
Carbohydrate	20.4%
Fat, total	47.1%
Alcohol	0.0%

Vitamins & Minerals		
Sodium	1060.037	mg
Potassium	561.202	mg
Vitamin A (RE)	329.425	RE
Vitamin C	23.889	mg
Calcium	128.400	mg
Iron	4.706	mg
Vitamin D (ug)	0.000	µg
Thiamin	0.079	mg
Riboflavin	0.230	mg
Niacin	5.501	mg
Pyridoxine (Vitamin B6)	0.349	mg
Folate (Total)	19.611	µg
Cobalamin (Vitamin B12)	1.675	µg
Biotin	0.306	µg
Pantothenic Acid	0.919	mg
Vitamin K	311.039	µg
Phosphorus	232.371	mg
Magnesium	61.297	mg
Zinc	5.479	mg
Copper	0.178	mg
Manganese	0.337	mg
Selenium	17.143	µg
Chromium	0.007	mg

Preheat oven to 400ºF. Cut the squash in half and scoop out the seeds. Place squash on a parchment paper–lined baking pan face down, and bake until soft, about 45–55 minutes. While the spaghetti squash is baking, prepare meat sauce.

In a large skillet, sauté onion and garlic in oil over medium heat for 3–5 minutes. Add ground beef and seasonings, and sauté until only a small amount of pink color remains. Add diced tomatoes, cover, reduce heat to low, and simmer for 15–20 minutes to allow flavors to combine. Add chard, stir, cover again, and remove from heat.

Scoop spaghetti squash meat from the shells, and divide between 4 bowls. Top with warm meat sauce and serve. Serves 4.

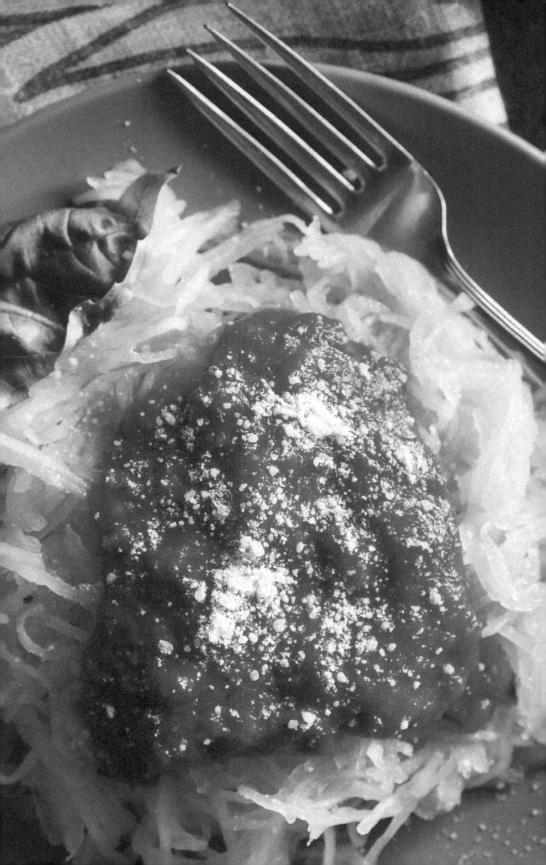

CHICKEN MARSALA

INGREDIENTS

1½ pounds skinless, boneless
chicken breasts (about 4 breasts)

2 tablespoons pumpkin seeds,
ground

2 tablespoons sunflower seeds,
ground

salt to taste

pepper to taste

¼ cup coconut oil

1 cup shiitake mushrooms,
stemmed and sliced

½ cup crimini mushrooms,
stemmed and sliced

½ cup sweet Marsala wine

½ cup chicken stock

2 tablespoons unsalted butter

¾ cup chopped flat-leaf parsley

4 cups kale, stems removed,
chopped

chopped fresh parsley, for garnish

Macronutrients		
Kilocalories	495.661	kcal
Trans Fatty Acid		g
Sugar, Total		g
Protein	44.838	g
Carbohydrate	11.064	g
Fat, Total	28.882	g
Alcohol	3.116	g
Cholesterol	139.161	mg
Saturated Fat	16.927	g
Monounsaturated Fat	4.917	g
Polyunsaturated Fat	3.308	g
Trans Fatty Acid	0.247	g
Dietary Fiber, Total	4.104	g
Sugar, Total	2.961	g

Percentage of Kcals	
Protein	35.5%
Carbohydrate	8.8%
Fat, total	51.4%
Alcohol	4.3%

Vitamins & Minerals		
Sodium	264.435	mg
Potassium	1075.415	mg
Vitamin A (RE)	826.986	RE
Vitamin C	95.707	mg
Calcium	137.268	mg
Iron	3.162	mg
Vitamin D (ug)	0.214	µg
Thiamin	0.290	mg
Riboflavin	0.513	mg
Niacin	15.918	mg
Pyridoxine (Vitamin B6)	1.462	mg
Folate (Total)	140.263	µg
Cobalamin (Vitamin B12)	0.256	µg
Biotin	0.176	µg
Pantothenic Acid	3.285	mg
Vitamin K	660.514	µg
Phosphorus	490.394	mg
Magnesium	122.861	mg
Zinc	2.640	mg
Copper	1.320	mg
Manganese	0.873	mg
Selenium	46.737	µg
Chromium	0.002	mg

Prepare chicken by tenderizing it. Place the meat between two layers of plastic wrap, and pound it with a meat mallet. You can also use the back of a large wooden spoon. Pound until the chicken breasts are about ¼ inch thick. In a separate bowl, combine ground seeds with salt and pepper.

Heat the coconut oil over medium to high heat in a large skillet. Dredge the chicken breasts on all sides in the seed mixture, and transfer them to the skillet. Fry the chicken breasts for about 3–5 minutes per side. You can do this in batches if all the chicken won't fit into the pan. Place the chicken on a baking pan in a single layer, and cover with a towel or place in a warm oven to keep warm.

Lower the heat to medium-low, add mushrooms, and sauté until moisture has evaporated. Season with more salt and pepper if desired. Pour Marsala wine into the pan, and allow alcohol to cook off, about 5 minutes. Add chicken broth and simmer for another 5 minutes. Stir in the butter, add the chicken breasts, and simmer gently for 1–3 minutes until chicken is warmed. Serve over kale, and top with fresh parsley.

Serves 4.

SLOW-COOKER BEEF BRISKET

INGREDIENTS

1 5-pound beef brisket (organic and grass fed if possible)

1 cup finely chopped yellow onion

½ cup water

3 tablespoons apple cider vinegar

2 tablespoons tamari

1 teaspoon garlic powder

1 teaspoon onion powder

1 teaspoon freshly ground black pepper

¼ teaspoon ground ginger

¼ teaspoon ground mustard powder

¼ teaspoon cinnamon

For the spice rub:

3 tablespoons paprika

1 tablespoon chili powder

1 tablespoon ground cumin

1 tablespoon kosher salt

1 teaspoon freshly ground black pepper

1 teaspoon cayenne pepper

1 teaspoon garlic powder

1 teaspoon onion powder

Macronutrients		
Kilocalories	192.254	kcal
Trans Fatty Acid		g
Sugar, Total		g
Protein	26.498	g
Carbohydrate	7.621	g
Fat, Total	6.730	g
Alcohol	0.000	g
Cholesterol	75.978	mg
Saturated Fat	2.229	g
Monounsaturated Fat	3.225	g
Polyunsaturated Fat	0.681	g
Trans Fatty Acid	0.229	g
Dietary Fiber, Total	2.916	g
Sugar, Total	1.689	g
Percentage of Kcals		
Protein	53.8%	
Carbohydrate	15.5%	
Fat, total	30.7%	
Alcohol	0.0%	
Vitamins & Minerals		
Sodium	1449.968	mg
Potassium	609.609	mg
Vitamin A (RE)	220.567	RE
Vitamin C	2.419	mg
Calcium	51.784	mg
Iron	3.620	mg
Vitamin D (ug)	0.113	µg
Vitamin E (mg)	0.159	mg
Thiamin	0.120	mg
Riboflavin	0.251	mg
Niacin	7.755	mg
Pyridoxine (Vitamin B6)	0.862	mg
Folate (Total)	11.715	µg
Cobalamin (Vitamin B12)	2.053	µg
Biotin	0.297	µg
Pantothenic Acid	0.968	mg
Vitamin K	7.161	µg
Phosphorus	282.309	mg
Magnesium	41.594	mg
Zinc	6.231	mg
Copper	0.148	mg
Manganese	0.284	mg
Selenium	28.930	µg
Chromium	0.009	mg

Combine ingredients for the spice rub. Cut brisket in half widthwise, and massage the rub into all areas of the brisket. Wrap in plastic wrap and refrigerate for at least 12 hours. Combine all remaining ingredients in the slow cooker, and stir to combine. Add brisket, and cook on low for about 10–12 hours until brisket is fork tender. Serve over coleslaw (recipe on page 89).

Serves 6.

Recipe Tidbit:

If you don't have time to allow the brisket to marinate in the spice rub for a full 12 hours, don't worry. The slow cooker will cause the flavors to mingle nicely. Whenever I am using a recipe that requires a spice rub, I double the recipe and save half in an airtight container for later use. It speeds things up nicely next time you need the same rub.

SLOW-COOKER TACO MEAT

INGREDIENTS

1 pound ground beef

1 24-ounce jar salsa (sugar-free) with your desired level of spiciness

1 onion, minced

4 cloves garlic, minced

2 large carrots, minced

1 teaspoon chili powder

1 teaspoon paprika

1 teaspoon onion powder

1 teaspoon garlic powder

½ teaspoon cumin

¼ teaspoon crushed red pepper flakes

salt and black pepper to taste

Macronutrients		
Kilocalories	194.746	kcal
Trans Fatty Acid		g
Sugar, Total		g
Protein	17.183	g
Carbohydrate	12.663	g
Fat, Total	8.126	g
Alcohol	0.000	g
Cholesterol	48.398	mg
Saturated Fat	2.669	g
Monounsaturated Fat	2.915	g
Polyunsaturated Fat	0.335	g
Trans Fatty Acid	0.408	g
Dietary Fiber, Total	3.533	g
Sugar, Total	5.840	g

Percentage of Kcals	
Protein	35.7%
Carbohydrate	26.3%
Fat, total	38.0%
Alcohol	0.0%

Vitamins & Minerals		
Sodium	759.007	mg
Potassium	666.819	mg
Vitamin A (RE)	425.258	RE
Vitamin C	17.279	mg
Calcium	39.546	mg
Iron	2.759	mg
Vitamin D (ug)	0.075	µg
Thiamin	0.103	mg
Riboflavin	0.184	mg
Niacin	5.615	mg
Pyridoxine (Vitamin B6)	0.337	mg
Folate (Total)	20.469	µg
Cobalamin (Vitamin B12)	1.253	µg
Biotin	0.814	µg
Pantothenic Acid	0.738	mg
Vitamin K	19.634	µg
Phosphorus	206.768	mg
Magnesium	43.576	mg
Zinc	4.072	mg
Copper	0.180	mg
Manganese	0.294	mg
Selenium	14.131	µg
Chromium	0.005	mg
Molybdenum	1.757	µg

Place all ingredients in the slow cooker, and stir to combine. Cook on low for 6–8 hours.

Serves 6.

Recipe Tidbit:

This is very easy to throw together in the morning. Then you come home to a meal that is almost ready. I serve it over greens for a taco salad. You could also serve the meat on jicama chips (see page 136) or rolled up in collard greens and baked in enchilada sauce. As I've said elsewhere, use this recipe and the others in the book to help you broaden your thinking when preparing meals.

PULLED CHICKEN

INGREDIENTS

1½ pounds boneless, skinless chicken breast (about 4 chicken breasts)

1 onion, minced

5 cloves garlic, minced

½ cup water

2 tablespoons apple cider vinegar

2 tablespoons tomato paste

1 tablespoon yellow mustard

1 teaspoon garlic powder

1 teaspoon onion powder

1 teaspoon salt

½ teaspoon cumin

4 cups kale, stems removed, chopped

4 cups mixed greens

Macronutrients		
Kilocalories	272.605	kcal
Trans Fatty Acid		g
Sugar, Total		g
Protein	42.998	g
Carbohydrate	13.832	g
Fat, Total	5.151	g
Alcohol	0.000	g
Cholesterol	123.896	mg
Saturated Fat	0.980	g
Monounsaturated Fat	1.165	g
Polyunsaturated Fat	0.995	g
Trans Fatty Acid	0.012	g
Dietary Fiber, Total	4.382	g
Sugar, Total	4.079	g
Percentage of Kcals		
Protein	62.8%	
Carbohydrate	20.2%	
Fat, total	16.9%	
Alcohol	0.0%	
Vitamins & Minerals		
Sodium	785.258	mg
Potassium	1070.095	mg
Vitamin A (RE)	741.609	RE
Vitamin C	89.006	mg
Calcium	154.124	mg
Iron	2.317	mg
Vitamin D (ug)	0.000	µg
Vitamin E (mg)	0.363	mg
Thiamin	0.245	mg
Riboflavin	0.411	mg
Niacin	14.203	mg
Pyridoxine (Vitamin B6)	1.419	mg
Folate (Total)	149.583	µg
Cobalamin (Vitamin B12)	0.232	µg
Biotin	0.863	µg
Pantothenic Acid	2.876	mg
Vitamin K	519.392	µg
Phosphorus	393.881	mg
Magnesium	84.896	mg
Zinc	1.949	mg
Copper	1.182	mg
Manganese	0.715	mg
Selenium	41.987	µg
Chromium	0.008	mg
Molybdenum	0.338	µg

Combine all ingredients except kale and mixed greens in a slow cooker, and stir to combine. Cook on low for 10–12 hours until chicken is tender. Transfer the breasts to a cutting board; using two forks, tease the meat apart. Return chicken to the slow cooker, and stir to combine.

Divide the greens between 4 serving bowls, and top with chicken mixture.

Serves 4.

Recipe Tidbit:

For a bit more flavor and fat (which increases satiety), you could top the chicken mixture with a light salad dressing.

COLLARD GREEN ROLL-UPS

INGREDIENTS

4 large collard green leaves

1 pound cooked chicken, chilled
   and sliced into long strips

1 cucumber, sliced into long strips

1 avocado, sliced into long strips

1 large carrot, peeled and sliced
   into long, thin strips

salt and pepper to taste

For the sauce (optional):

2 cloves garlic, minced

3 tablespoons green salsa

2 tablespoons lime juice

1 tablespoon olive oil

1 tablespoon water

salt and pepper to taste

Macronutrients		
Kilocalories	283.116	kcal
Trans Fatty Acid		g
Sugar, Total		g
Protein	34.538	g
Carbohydrate	8.880	g
Fat, Total	12.121	g
Alcohol	0.000	g
Cholesterol	87.317	mg
Saturated Fat	2.176	g
Monounsaturated Fat	6.912	g
Polyunsaturated Fat	1.758	g
Trans Fatty Acid	0.000	g
Dietary Fiber, Total	3.298	g
Sugar, Total	2.396	g
Percentage of Kcals		
Protein	48.9%	
Carbohydrate	12.6%	
Fat, total	38.6%	
Alcohol	0.0%	
Vitamins & Minerals		
Sodium	153.029	mg
Potassium	556.009	mg
Vitamin A (RE)	289.619	RE
Vitamin C	10.509	mg
Calcium	46.382	mg
Iron	1.653	mg
Vitamin D (ug)	0.113	µg
Thiamin	0.108	mg
Riboflavin	0.219	mg
Niacin	10.488	mg
Pyridoxine (Vitamin B6)	0.543	mg
Folate (Total)	42.126	µg
Cobalamin (Vitamin B12)	0.261	µg
Biotin	0.458	µg
Pantothenic Acid	1.394	mg
Vitamin K	23.703	µg
Phosphorus	231.925	mg
Magnesium	49.548	mg
Zinc	1.538	mg
Copper	0.150	mg
Manganese	0.178	mg
Selenium	25.883	µg
Chromium	0.001	mg
Molybdenum	1.317	µg

Whisk together ingredients for the sauce, if using. Set aside.

Pour about 2 inches of water into a large saucepan, and bring to a low simmer over medium-high heat. Submerge 1 leaf of collard greens in the water to blanch, just long enough to allow it to soften and turn bright green, about 1 minute. Remove from the pan, pat dry, and set aside. Repeat the process for the remaining 3 leaves. Now you are ready to assemble the roll-ups. Divide the chicken, cucumber, avocado, and carrot evenly between the 4 collard green leaves, sprinkle with salt and pepper, and form into a roll. Top with sauce if desired. Serve immediately.

Recipe tidbit:

For an even easier version, replace the chicken with store-bought cold cuts. Make sure they are sugar- and nitrite-free. Or try eggs: Lightly fry beaten eggs in a small pan, flipping them like an omelet. Remove from heat, and cut into thin strips to add to your wraps. You could also experiment with using many different types of vegetable.

GARLIC BUFFALO MEATBALLS

INGREDIENTS

1 tablespoon olive oil

1 pound ground buffalo

1 tablespoon ground pumpkin seeds

1 tablespoon ground sunflower seeds

½ tablespoon ground flaxseeds

2 eggs, lightly beaten with a fork

1 tablespoon plus 1 teaspoon minced garlic

1 tablespoon dried basil

1 tablespoon dried oregano

1 tablespoon dried parsley

1 tablespoon garlic powder

1 teaspoon dried rosemary, crushed

1 teaspoon dried marjoram

1 teaspoon salt

½ teaspoon pepper

6 cups kale, stems removed, chopped

6 cups mixed greens

Macronutrients		
Kilocalories	191.862	kcal
Trans Fatty Acid		g
Sugar, Total		g
Protein	23.362	g
Carbohydrate	11.084	g
Fat, Total	7.475	g
Alcohol	0.000	g
Cholesterol	62.000	mg
Saturated Fat	1.502	g
Monounsaturated Fat	3.150	g
Polyunsaturated Fat	1.597	g
Trans Fatty Acid	0.056	g
Dietary Fiber, Total	4.594	g
Sugar, Total	2.029	g
Percentage of Kcals		
Protein	45.6%	
Carbohydrate	21.6%	
Fat, total	32.8%	
Alcohol	0.0%	
Vitamins & Minerals		
Sodium	479.569	mg
Potassium	828.799	mg
Vitamin A (RE)	757.429	RE
Vitamin C	84.905	mg
Calcium	178.830	mg
Iron	5.038	mg
Vitamin D (ug)	0.333	µg
Vitamin E (mg)	0.538	mg
Thiamin	0.258	mg
Riboflavin	0.464	mg
Niacin	6.366	mg
Pyridoxine (Vitamin B6)	0.913	mg
Folate (Total)	151.427	µg
Cobalamin (Vitamin B12)	1.018	µg
Biotin	0.557	µg
Pantothenic Acid	1.145	mg
Vitamin K	539.958	µg
Phosphorus	300.036	mg
Magnesium	81.472	mg
Zinc	3.412	mg
Copper	1.244	mg
Manganese	0.856	mg
Selenium	12.650	µg
Chromium	0.004	mg
Molybdenum	0.338	µg

Preheat oven to 350ºF. Grease a 13 x 9–inch baking dish with 1 table-spoon olive oil; place dish in the oven while oven is heating. Place buffalo, seeds, eggs, and seasonings in a medium mixing bowl. Mix well with hands to combine into a uniform mixture. Form into 12 meatballs. Arrange in baking dish. Bake for 15 minutes; turn meatballs, and continue baking for about 10 more minutes or until browned and cooked to your desired level of doneness.

Serve warm over 2 cups of greens per person.

Serves 6.

Recipe Tidbit:

Substitute leftover cooked brown rice for the ground seeds if you desire. Use about 3–4 tablespoons of rice, mashed first.

To serve, top with any sauce you desire as long as it doesn't contain sugar. Alternatively, if you get used to eating foods like this without added sauce or salad dressing, you cut down on calories and get used to the foods' real flavors.

MAKIZUSHI (SUSHI ROLLS)

Restaurant sushi is expensive and always contains sugar and white rice, both of which are terrible for keeping blood sugar well regulated. Here is a fun and easy way to make your own sushi rolls at home. You can do some amazing things without rice.

INGREDIENTS

1 cucumber, peeled and cut into long, thin strips

8 ounces smoked salmon (no sugar added), cut into long strips

8 green onions, green part only

5 avocados, mashed

1 teaspoon toasted sesame seeds

8 sheets toasted seaweed

wheat-free tamari for dipping

wasabi paste, to be added to tamari dipping sauce

Macronutrients		
Kilocalories	567.538	kcal
Trans Fatty Acid		g
Sugar, Total		g
Protein	29.050	g
Carbohydrate	21.545	g
Fat, Total	43.220	g
Alcohol	0.000	g
Cholesterol	60.669	mg
Saturated Fat	7.587	g
Monounsaturated Fat	26.089	g
Polyunsaturated Fat	3.420	g
Trans Fatty Acid	0.000	g
Dietary Fiber, Total	14.632	g
Sugar, Total	2.460	g
Percentage of Kcals		
Protein	19.6%	
Carbohydrate	14.6%	
Fat, total	65.8%	
Alcohol	0.0%	
Vitamins & Minerals		
Sodium	412.864	mg
Potassium	1440.233	mg
Vitamin A (RE)	230.070	RE
Vitamin C	27.252	mg
Calcium	69.278	mg
Iron	4.997	mg
Vitamin D (ug)	0.000	µg
Thiamin	0.204	mg
Riboflavin	0.450	mg
Niacin	10.153	mg
Pyridoxine (Vitamin B6)	0.529	mg
Folate (Total)	173.829	µg
Cobalamin (Vitamin B12)	0.000	µg
Biotin	1.200	µg
Pantothenic Acid	2.667	mg
Vitamin K	109.533	µg
Phosphorus	124.555	mg
Magnesium	66.549	mg
Zinc	1.472	mg
Copper	0.350	mg
Manganese	0.366	mg
Selenium	1.303	µg
Chromium	0.006	mg

Special equipment: 1 sushi roller and paddle (available at Asian grocers for under $5).

Place one sheet of seaweed on the sushi roller, making sure to arrange the sheet so that the perforation will aid in cutting the roll once you assemble it. Place the seaweed sheet rough side up (i.e., so it will be in contact with the avocado).

Spoon a small amount of avocado onto seaweed sheet, and pat it flat with the sushi paddle, leaving a border of ½–1 inch without avocado at the top edge (i.e., the edge farthest away from you) of the seaweed sheet. Place 1–2 strips each of cucumber, smoked salmon, and green onion on top of the avocado at the bottom edge of the seaweed sheet. Use the sushi roller to roll it up, like a jelly roll. With a very sharp, serrated, clean knife, cut the roll into ¾-inch makizushi, or sushi rolls.

Helpful hints: As with anything, learning to make sushi rolls can take a little practice. Your earliest rolls will still taste great, however, so use them as "tasters" until you have a better handle on the technique.

Clean the knife between each roll for easier slicing. Allow yourself plenty of time to get the feel of it. Sometimes using less avocado and fewer vegetables can make it easier to roll.

Serve immediately. Each person should get his or her own sauce dish to mix tamari and wasabi to desired taste.

Serves 4.

Recipe Tidbit:

Sushi rolls are very fun to experiment with. Sprinkle the avocado with toasted sesame seeds before rolling. Ideas for veggies include radishes, jicama, bok choy, sprouts, or pickles. Another way of making grain-free sushi is to use finely chopped steamed cauliflower in place of rice.

STEAK WRAPS WITH CHIMICHURRI SAUCE

Contrary to what you may think, in this recipe the steak is wrapped around delicious vegetables.

INGREDIENTS

1 pound sirloin or flank steak, cut into 8 thin slices

1 tablespoon butter

1 tablespoon balsamic vinegar

salt and pepper to taste

1 tablespoon olive oil

1 red bell pepper, cut into long strips

1 green bell pepper, cut into long strips

2 medium zucchinis, center seeds removed, cut into long strips

1 large carrot, peeled and cut into long strips

Chimichurri sauce:

1 cup (packed) fresh Italian parsley

½ cup olive oil

⅓ cup red wine vinegar

¼ cup (packed) fresh cilantro

2 garlic cloves, peeled

1 teaspoon lemon juice

¾ teaspoon crushed red pepper

½ teaspoon ground cumin

½ teaspoon salt

Macronutrients		
Kilocalories	537.112	kcal
Trans Fatty Acid		g
Sugar, Total		g
Protein	27.158	g
Carbohydrate	10.588	g
Fat, Total	42.890	g
Alcohol	0.000	g
Cholesterol	60.521	mg
Saturated Fat	9.974	g
Monounsaturated Fat	27.356	g
Polyunsaturated Fat	3.865	g
Trans Fatty Acid	0.400	g
Dietary Fiber, Total	3.294	g
Sugar, Total	5.350	g

Percentage of Kcals	
Protein	20.2%
Carbohydrate	7.9%
Fat, total	71.9%
Alcohol	0.0%

Vitamins & Minerals		
Sodium	417.606	mg
Potassium	899.045	mg
Vitamin A (RE)	547.517	RE
Vitamin C	101.885	mg
Calcium	61.512	mg
Iron	3.937	mg
Vitamin D (ug)	0.190	µg
Vitamin E (mg)	0.083	mg
Thiamin	0.230	mg
Riboflavin	0.473	mg
Niacin	9.036	mg
Pyridoxine (Vitamin B6)	0.647	mg
Folate (Total)	72.615	µg
Cobalamin (Vitamin B12)	2.852	µg
Biotin	0.458	µg
Pantothenic Acid	1.234	mg
Vitamin K	279.441	µg
Phosphorus	300.205	mg
Magnesium	64.487	mg
Zinc	7.636	mg
Copper	0.228	mg
Manganese	0.344	mg
Selenium	33.989	µg
Chromium	0.009	mg
Molybdenum	1.317	µg

Prepare chimichurri sauce by combining all ingredients in a food processor or blender and processing to the consistency of a chunky sauce.

Warm butter just to liquid consistency, and whisk together with balsamic vinegar. Generously brush butter–balsamic mixture onto steak pieces, sprinkle with salt and pepper, and set aside.

Sauté all vegetables in olive oil over medium heat until crisp tender. Sprinkle with salt and pepper to taste. Set aside. Cook steak in a frying pan over medium heat for 1–2 minutes on each side, or to your desired level of doneness. Remove promptly, and arrange sautéed vegetables on top of steak slices. Roll up, steak side out, securing each wrap with a toothpick. Serve with chimichurri sauce.

Serves 4.

ZA'ATAR SPICED CHICKEN

INGREDIENTS

1 whole organic chicken, 5–6
pounds

1 orange, halved

1 lemon, halved

2 tablespoons + 1 tablespoon butter
melted

1 white or yellow onion, chopped

4 large carrots, peeled and chopped

2 celery stalks, chopped

salt and pepper to taste

For the rub:

3 tablespoons dried thyme

2 tablespoons toasted sesame seeds

2 tablespoons marjoram

2 tablespoons oregano

1 tablespoon sumac spice

1 teaspoon onion powder

1 teaspoon garlic powder

1 teaspoon salt

Macronutrients		
Kilocalories	323.572	kcal
Protein	24.207	g
Carbohydrate	8.208	g
Fat, Total	22.201	g
Alcohol	0.000	g
Cholesterol	133.068	mg
Saturated Fat	7.571	g
Monounsaturated Fat	9.254	g
Polyunsaturated Fat	3.827	g
Trans Fatty Acid	0.359	g
Dietary Fiber, Total	3.108	g
Sugar, Total	2.489	g
Percentage of Kcals		
Protein	29.4%	
Carbohydrate	10.0%	
Fat, total	60.6%	
Alcohol	0.0%	
Vitamins & Minerals		
Sodium	440.603	mg
Potassium	592.991	mg
Vitamin A (RE)	596.052	RE
Vitamin C	6.365	mg
Calcium	92.013	mg
Iron	3.923	mg
Vitamin D (ug)	0.817	µg
Vitamin E (mg)	0.308	mg
Thiamin	0.199	mg
Riboflavin	0.351	mg
Niacin	8.372	mg
Pyridoxine (Vitamin B6)	0.479	mg
Folate (Total)	34.959	µg
Cobalamin (Vitamin B12)	0.009	µg
Biotin	2.944	µg
Pantothenic Acid	1.403	mg
Vitamin K	45.590	µg
Phosphorus	209.593	mg
Magnesium	49.219	mg
Zinc	1.786	mg
Copper	0.143	mg
Manganese	0.417	mg
Selenium	15.933	µg
Chromium	0.022	mg
Molybdenum	2.802	µg

Combine all ingredients for the rub. Set aside.

Remove the chicken giblets, rinse the chicken inside and out, and remove any excess fat. Pat the outside of the chicken dry, stuff center cavity with lemon and orange halves, and massage the rub mixture generously onto the skin of the entire chicken. Wrap in plastic wrap, and refrigerate for at least 12 hours to allow flavors to mingle.

Preheat the oven to 425°F. Brush the outside of the chicken with

2 tablespoons butter, and sprinkle again with salt and pepper. Tie the legs together with kitchen string, and tuck the wing tips under the body. Place the onions, carrots, and celery in a roasting pan, and toss with a small amount of salt and 1 tablespoon butter. Place the chicken on top of the vegetables, and roast for 80–100 minutes or until juices run clear when you cut between a leg and a thigh. If you want to use a meat thermometer, roast the chicken until the temperature reaches 160°F at the thickest part of the thigh. Remove chicken from the oven, tent loosely with foil, and allow to rest on the roasting pan for 10 minutes or until the internal temperature reaches 165°F.

Cut the chicken into pieces, and serve with the roasted vegetables.

Serves 8.

ASIAN ZUCCHINI NOODLES

INGREDIENTS

2 tablespoons + 1 tablespoon olive oil

½ cup onion, minced small

3 cloves garlic

1 teaspoon minced fresh ginger, peeled first

1 teaspoon lemongrass paste (optional)

4 small zucchinis, worked into spirals or straight sticks (see below)

1 cup cubed cooked chicken, chilled

2 eggs, lightly beaten

2 tablespoons water

1 teaspoon gluten-free tamari

1 teaspoon sugar-free fish sauce

1 teaspoon fresh lime juice

1 teaspoon ground white pepper

red pepper flakes to taste (optional)

salt to taste

fresh cilantro, for garnish

Macronutrients		
Kilocalories	471.466	kcal
Trans Fatty Acid		g
Sugar, Total		g
Protein	31.491	g
Carbohydrate	19.268	g
Fat, Total	31.054	g
Alcohol	0.000	g
Cholesterol	244.100	mg
Saturated Fat	6.007	g
Monounsaturated Fat	18.337	g
Polyunsaturated Fat	4.549	g
Trans Fatty Acid	0.019	g
Dietary Fiber, Total	5.039	g
Sugar, Total	11.896	g

Percentage of Kcals	
Protein	26.1%
Carbohydrate	16.0%
Fat, total	57.9%
Alcohol	0.0%

Vitamins & Minerals		
Sodium	553.679	mg
Potassium	1311.585	mg
Vitamin A (RE)	170.266	RE
Vitamin C	75.619	mg
Calcium	123.501	mg
Iron	3.682	mg
Vitamin D (ug)	1.070	µg
Vitamin E (mg)	0.526	mg
Thiamin	0.260	mg
Riboflavin	0.731	mg
Niacin	6.248	mg
Pyridoxine (Vitamin B6)	1.025	mg
Folate (Total)	131.532	µg
Cobalamin (Vitamin B12)	0.613	µg
Biotin	0.445	µg
Pantothenic Acid	2.173	mg
Vitamin K	31.129	µg
Phosphorus	374.467	mg
Magnesium	103.499	mg
Zinc	3.438	mg
Copper	0.332	mg
Manganese	0.909	mg
Selenium	31.923	µg
Chromium	0.018	mg

Use one of the following methods to prepare the zucchini: (1) use a food processer; (2) use an inexpensive (about $15) vegetable spiral slicer; (3) use a julienne peeler. The spiral slicer will give you spiral "noodles," and the julienne peeler will produce straight sticks.

Sauté the onion, garlic, ginger, and lemongrass paste (if you are using it) in 2 tablespoons olive oil for 3 minutes over medium heat. Toss in the zucchini and chicken, and sauté for another 3–5 minutes. Push mixture to the sides; add 1 tablespoon of oil and then the eggs. Cook until the eggs begin to get puffy; flip them over. Cook for a bit longer, then cut eggs into pieces in the pan and incorporate into the chicken mixture. Add the water, tamari, fish sauce, lime juice, white pepper, and red pepper flakes (if desired), and incorporate. Add salt to taste. Garnish with fresh cilantro.

Serve immediately.

Serves 2.

PESTO "PASTA"

INGREDIENTS

2 tablespoons olive oil

2 cloves garlic, minced

4 small zucchinis, worked into
spirals or straight sticks (see
page 156)

½ cup basil pesto (see recipe on
page 82)

2 cups arugula

1 pint cherry tomatoes, halved

fresh flat leaf parsley, chopped for
garnish

salt and pepper to taste

grated Parmesan cheese
(optional)

Macronutrients		
Kilocalories	449.479	kcal
Trans Fatty Acid		g
Sugar, Total		g
Protein	8.880	g
Carbohydrate	16.199	g
Fat, Total	39.436	g
Alcohol	0.000	g
Cholesterol	0.000	mg
Saturated Fat	5.310	g
Monounsaturated Fat	24.941	g
Polyunsaturated Fat	6.886	g
Trans Fatty Acid	0.000	g
Dietary Fiber, Total	5.084	g
Sugar, Total	15.724	g

Percentage of Kcals	
Protein	7.8%
Carbohydrate	14.2%
Fat, total	78.0%
Alcohol	0.0%

Vitamins & Minerals		
Sodium	160.321	mg
Potassium	1740.094	mg
Vitamin A (RE)	417.491	RE
Vitamin C	127.453	mg
Calcium	174.214	mg
Iron	4.022	mg
Vitamin D (ug)	0.000	µg
Vitamin E (mg)	2.075	mg
Thiamin	0.334	mg
Riboflavin	0.498	mg
Niacin	4.163	mg
Pyridoxine (Vitamin B6)	1.000	mg
Folate (Total)	164.757	µg
Cobalamin (Vitamin B12)	0.000	µg
Biotin	2.551	µg
Pantothenic Acid	1.424	mg
Vitamin K	181.447	µg
Phosphorus	278.187	mg
Magnesium	137.765	mg
Zinc	2.477	mg
Copper	0.553	mg
Manganese	2.020	mg
Selenium	1.628	µg
Chromium	0.010	mg

In a large skillet, sweat the garlic in olive oil for 3 minutes over medium-low heat. Increase heat to medium; add zucchini and pesto, and sauté until zucchini is cooked to your desired level of doneness (ideally, it will still have a little crunch). Toss in arugula and cherry tomatoes, stir to combine, and remove from heat. Serve topped with parsley, salt, pepper, and Parmesan if desired.

Serve immediately.

Serves 2.

Chapter 6
BEVERAGES

CARDAMOM COLD BREW

INGREDIENTS

1 ¾ cups coffee beans, coarsely
ground

3 ¾ cup filtered water

2½ cups unsweetened almond
milk

1 teaspoon ground cardamom

In a large airtight jar, combine
water with coffee; shake well, and
allow to sit on counter overnight
or for at least 12 hours. Shake the
mixture a few times during this
brewing period.

Next, gently pour off the liquid
through a coffee filter into a new

Macronutrients		
Kilocalories	47.429	kcal
Trans Fatty Acid		g
Sugar, Total		g
Protein	4.685	g
Carbohydrate	2.774	g
Fat, Total	2.301	g
Alcohol	0.000	g
Cholesterol	0.000	mg
Saturated Fat	0.255	g
Monounsaturated Fat	0.521	g
Polyunsaturated Fat	1.253	g
Trans Fatty Acid	0.000	g
Dietary Fiber, Total	2.112	g
Sugar, Total	0.500	g

Percentage of Kcals	
Protein	37.1%
Carbohydrate	22.0%
Fat, total	41.0%
Alcohol	0.0%

Vitamins & Minerals		
Sodium	17.442	mg
Potassium	212.541	mg
Vitamin A (RE)	0.000	RE
Vitamin C	0.084	mg
Calcium	24.193	mg
Iron	0.981	mg
Vitamin D (ug)	0.000	µg
Thiamin	0.017	mg
Riboflavin	0.091	mg
Niacin	0.231	mg
Pyridoxine (Vitamin B6)	0.002	mg
Folate (Total)	2.370	µg
Cobalamin (Vitamin B12)	0.000	µg
Pantothenic Acid	0.301	mg
Vitamin K	0.119	µg
Phosphorus	4.267	mg
Magnesium	4.471	mg
Zinc	0.054	mg
Copper	0.004	mg
Manganese	0.139	mg
Selenium	0.000	µg

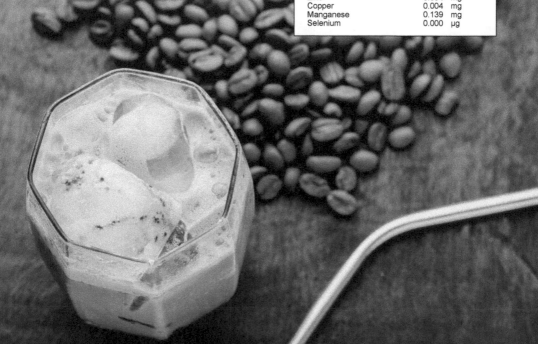

container. This should yield about 2½ cups of cold-brew concentrate. Mix with equal parts almond milk, usually about 2½ cups. Add cardamom, and shake gently. Chill in refrigerator. Shake well before each serving.

Recipe Tidbit:

You can make this recipe your own. For a creamier version, if you are able to tolerate dairy, add ½ cup organic half and half or heavy whipping cream. You can eliminate the cardamom or add other spices such as cinnamon. Try adding the spices to the coffee mixture while it is brewing. Cold brew is traditionally sweetened, but I think this recipe is fine the way it is. Depending on the coffee you use, it can turn out a little bitter, so pick a light to medium roast to reduce the bitterness. If the coffee is too strong, add extra almond milk to dilute.

ACV WATER

INGREDIENTS

24 fluid ounces (3 cups) filtered water
½ teaspoon apple cider vinegar

Combine ingredients, and enjoy.

Serves 1.

Recipe Tidbit:

This blend is one of my long-time favorites. It's what I usually have in my 24-ounce water bottle. The vinegar adds just enough flavor to make the water tasty. Be sure to buy an organic apple cider vinegar that contains "the mother"—the sediment at the bottom of the bottle. Shake the vinegar well before using.

Macronutrients		
Kilocalories	0.000	kcal
Trans Fatty Acid		g
Sugar, Total		g
Protein	0.000	g
Carbohydrate	0.000	g
Fat, Total	0.000	g
Alcohol	0.000	g
Cholesterol	0.000	mg
Saturated Fat	0.000	g
Monounsaturated Fat	0.000	g
Polyunsaturated Fat	0.000	g
Trans Fatty Acid	0.000	g
Dietary Fiber, Total	0.000	g
Sugar, Total	0.000	g

Percentage of Kcals	
Protein	0.0%
Carbohydrate	0.0%
Fat, total	0.0%
Alcohol	0.0%

Vitamins & Minerals		
Sodium	20.470	mg
Potassium	6.823	mg
Vitamin A (RE)	0.000	RE
Vitamin C	0.000	mg
Calcium	20.470	mg
Iron	0.000	mg
Vitamin D (ug)	0.000	µg
Thiamin	0.000	mg
Riboflavin	0.000	mg
Niacin	0.000	mg
Pyridoxine (Vitamin B6)	0.000	mg
Folate (Total)	0.000	µg
Cobalamin (Vitamin B12)	0.000	µg
Pantothenic Acid	0.000	mg
Vitamin K	0.000	µg
Phosphorus	0.000	mg
Magnesium	6.823	mg
Zinc	0.000	mg
Copper	0.060	mg
Manganese	0.000	mg
Selenium	0.000	µg

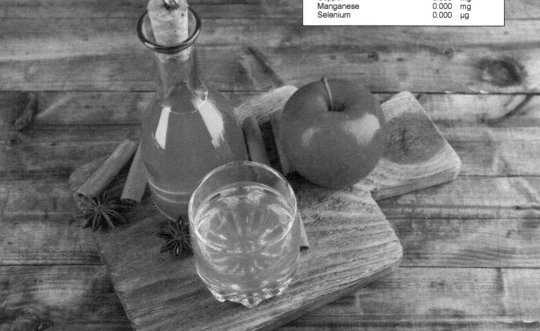

ACV APERITIF

INGREDIENTS

¼ to ½ cup filtered water

2 teaspoons apple cider vinegar

Combine ingredients. Ingest 20 minutes before a meal, especially a high-protein meal.

Serves 1.

Recipe Tidbit:

Consuming this drink will stimulate your digestion and help you digest proteins more easily. It's pretty tart, so I get it down fast.

Apple cider vinegar has been used for centuries for weight loss. Drink this concoction before each meal for 60 days, and you will notice a difference in your appetite and waistline.

Macronutrients		
Kilocalories	0.000	kcal
Trans Fatty Acid		g
Sugar, Total		g
Protein	0.000	g
Carbohydrate	0.000	g
Fat, Total	0.000	g
Alcohol	0.000	g
Cholesterol	0.000	mg
Saturated Fat	0.000	g
Monounsaturated Fat	0.000	g
Polyunsaturated Fat	0.000	g
Trans Fatty Acid	0.000	g
Dietary Fiber, Total	0.000	g
Sugar, Total	0.000	g

Percentage of Kcals	
Protein	0.0%
Carbohydrate	0.0%
Fat, total	0.0%
Alcohol	0.0%

Vitamins & Minerals		
Sodium	1.778	mg
Potassium	0.593	mg
Vitamin A (RE)	0.000	RE
Vitamin C	0.000	mg
Calcium	1.778	mg
Iron	0.000	mg
Vitamin D (ug)	0.000	µg
Thiamin	0.000	mg
Riboflavin	0.000	mg
Niacin	0.000	mg
Pyridoxine (Vitamin B6)	0.000	mg
Folate (Total)	0.000	µg
Cobalamin (Vitamin B12)	0.000	µg
Pantothenic Acid	0.000	µg
Vitamin K	0.000	µg
Phosphorus	0.000	mg
Magnesium	0.593	mg
Zinc	0.000	mg
Copper	0.005	mg
Manganese	0.000	mg
Selenium	0.000	µg

CUCUMBER WATER

INGREDIENTS

2 cups filtered water

½ cucumber, sliced

Add cucumbers to water and place in the refrigerator. Allow flavors to mingle for at least 30 minutes before serving. Serve chilled.

Serves 1.

Macronutrients		
Kilocalories	2.258	kcal
Trans Fatty Acid		g
Sugar, Total		g
Protein	0.098	g
Carbohydrate	0.546	g
Fat, Total	0.017	g
Alcohol	0.000	g
Cholesterol	0.000	mg
Saturated Fat	0.006	g
Monounsaturated Fat	0.001	g
Polyunsaturated Fat	0.005	g
Dietary Fiber, Total	0.075	g
Sugar, Total	0.251	g

Percentage of Kcals	
Protein	14.4%
Carbohydrate	80.2%
Fat, total	5.5%
Alcohol	0.0%

Vitamins & Minerals		
Sodium	14.521	mg
Potassium	26.864	mg
Vitamin A (RE)	1.580	RE
Vitamin C	0.421	mg
Calcium	16.628	mg
Iron	0.042	mg
Vitamin D (ug)	0.000	µg
Thiamin	0.004	mg
Riboflavin	0.005	mg
Niacin	0.015	mg
Pyridoxine (Vitamin B6)	0.006	mg
Folate (Total)	1.054	µg
Cobalamin (Vitamin B12)	0.000	µg
Pantothenic Acid	0.039	mg
Vitamin K	2.468	µg
Phosphorus	3.612	mg
Magnesium	6.697	mg
Zinc	0.030	mg
Copper	0.048	mg
Manganese	0.012	mg
Selenium	0.045	µg

SPARKLING LEMON WATER

INGREDIENTS

2 cups sparkling water

½ teaspoon fresh lemon juice

Add the lemon juice to the sparkling water and enjoy.

Serves 1.

Recipe Tidbit:

If you have a carbonator at home, you can make your own sparkling water. Otherwise, you can easily buy nonsweetened or flavored sparkling water. Because drinking plain water can get a little boring when you are supposed to drink ½ your weight in ounces of water daily, sparkling water enhanced with a nonsweetened flavoring can be a great alternative to plain water.

Macronutrients		
Kilocalories	0.559	kcal
Trans Fatty Acid		g
Sugar, Total		g
Protein	0.009	g
Carbohydrate	0.175	g
Fat, Total	0.006	g
Alcohol	0.000	g
Cholesterol	0.000	mg
Saturated Fat	0.001	g
Monounsaturated Fat	0.000	g
Polyunsaturated Fat	0.001	g
Trans Fatty Acid	0.000	g
Dietary Fiber, Total	0.008	g
Sugar, Total	0.064	g

Percentage of Kcals	
Protein	4.5%
Carbohydrate	88.6%
Fat, total	6.9%
Alcohol	0.0%

Vitamins & Minerals		
Sodium	0.025	mg
Potassium	2.618	mg
Vitamin A (RE)	0.015	RE
Vitamin C	0.984	mg
Calcium	0.153	mg
Iron	0.002	mg
Vitamin D (ug)	0.000	µg
Thiamin	0.001	mg
Riboflavin	0.000	mg
Niacin	0.002	mg
Pyridoxine (Vitamin B6)	0.001	mg
Folate (Total)	0.508	µg
Cobalamin (Vitamin B12)	0.000	µg
Pantothenic Acid	0.003	mg
Vitamin K	0.000	µg
Phosphorus	0.203	mg
Magnesium	0.153	mg
Zinc	0.001	mg
Copper	0.000	mg
Manganese	0.000	mg
Selenium	0.003	µg

HOT WATER WITH LEMON

INGREDIENTS

2 cups filtered water

2–4 slices of lemon or ½ teaspoon
fresh lemon juice

Warm the water in a saucepan over medium heat; remove from heat and pour into 2 separate glasses. Add lemon juice or lemon slices, and serve immediately.

Serves 2.

Recipe Tidbit:

This is a fabulous drink to consume daily throughout the winter. It keeps you warm and stimulates digestion. Drink this beverage about ½ hour before a meal to both stimulate digestion and control appetite. You can also order this beverage at a restaurant.

Macronutrients		
Kilocalories	0.280	kcal
Trans Fatty Acid		g
Sugar, Total		g
Protein	0.004	g
Carbohydrate	0.088	g
Fat, Total	0.003	g
Alcohol	0.000	g
Cholesterol	0.000	mg
Saturated Fat	0.001	g
Monounsaturated Fat	0.000	g
Polyunsaturated Fat	0.000	g
Trans Fatty Acid	0.000	g
Dietary Fiber, Total	0.004	g
Sugar, Total	0.032	g

Percentage of Kcals	
Protein	4.5%
Carbohydrate	88.6%
Fat, total	6.9%
Alcohol	0.0%

Vitamins & Minerals		
Sodium	7.123	mg
Potassium	3.679	mg
Vitamin A (RE)	0.008	RE
Vitamin C	0.492	mg
Calcium	7.186	mg
Iron	0.001	mg
Vitamin D (ug)	0.000	µg
Thiamin	0.000	mg
Riboflavin	0.000	mg
Niacin	0.001	mg
Pyridoxine (Vitamin B6)	0.001	mg
Folate (Total)	0.254	µg
Cobalamin (Vitamin B12)	0.000	µg
Pantothenic Acid	0.002	mg
Vitamin K	0.000	µg
Phosphorus	0.102	mg
Magnesium	2.446	mg
Zinc	0.001	mg
Copper	0.021	mg
Manganese	0.000	mg
Selenium	0.001	µg

WATER WITH MINT AND LIME

INGREDIENTS

4 cups filtered water

1 cup mint leaves

1 teaspoon lime juice

Combine all ingredients, and store in the refrigerator until use. Serve at room temperature or chilled.

Serves 2.

Macronutrients

Kilocalories	1.537	kcal
Trans Fatty Acid		g
Sugar, Total		g
Protein	0.059	g
Carbohydrate	0.407	g
Fat, Total	0.014	g
Alcohol	0.000	g
Cholesterol	0.000	mg
Saturated Fat	0.003	g
Monounsaturated Fat	0.001	g
Polyunsaturated Fat	0.007	g
Dietary Fiber, Total	0.113	g
Sugar, Total	0.043	g

Percentage of Kcals

Protein	11.8%
Carbohydrate	81.9%
Fat, total	6.3%
Alcohol	0.0%

Vitamins & Minerals

Sodium	14.668	mg
Potassium	15.021	mg
Vitamin A (RE)	5.562	RE
Vitamin C	1.177	mg
Calcium	17.688	mg
Iron	0.067	mg
Vitamin D (ug)	0.000	µg
Thiamin	0.002	mg
Riboflavin	0.004	mg
Niacin	0.025	mg
Pyridoxine (Vitamin B6)	0.003	mg
Folate (Total)	1.715	µg
Cobalamin (Vitamin B12)	0.000	µg
Pantothenic Acid	0.007	mg
Vitamin K	0.015	µg
Phosphorus	1.293	mg
Magnesium	5.969	mg
Zinc	0.016	mg
Copper	0.047	mg
Manganese	0.016	mg
Selenium	0.003	µg

KALE SMOOTHIE DELIGHT

INGREDIENTS

2 cups kale, stems removed and
  chopped

3 cups filtered water

½ teaspoon lime juice

1 cup frozen blackberries

Blend all ingredients in a high-powered blender until smooth.

Serves 2.

Recipe Tidbit:

I usually prefer my "green drinks" to
be green in color; the deep purple of
this tangy smoothie is a delightful
exception. Using red berries will
tend to turn it more brown, so stick
with blackberries.

Macronutrients		
Kilocalories	81.468	kcal
Trans Fatty Acid		g
Sugar, Total		g
Protein	3.764	g
Carbohydrate	17.801	g
Fat, Total	0.949	g
Alcohol	0.000	g
Cholesterol	0.000	mg
Saturated Fat	0.072	g
Monounsaturated Fat	0.066	g
Polyunsaturated Fat	0.412	g
Dietary Fiber, Total	6.192	g
Sugar, Total	9.591	g

Percentage of Kcals	
Protein	15.9%
Carbohydrate	75.1%
Fat, total	9.0%
Alcohol	0.0%

Vitamins & Minerals		
Sodium	36.906	mg
Potassium	439.720	mg
Vitamin A (RE)	677.698	RE
Vitamin C	83.125	mg
Calcium	133.238	mg
Iron	1.590	mg
Vitamin D (ug)	0.000	µg
Vitamin E (mg)	0.536	mg
Thiamin	0.096	mg
Riboflavin	0.122	mg
Niacin	1.583	mg
Pyridoxine (Vitamin B6)	0.228	mg
Folate (Total)	120.267	µg
Cobalamin (Vitamin B12)	0.000	µg
Pantothenic Acid	0.177	mg
Vitamin K	487.172	µg
Phosphorus	84.468	mg
Magnesium	51.757	mg
Zinc	0.565	mg
Copper	1.127	mg
Manganese	1.365	mg
Selenium	0.906	µg

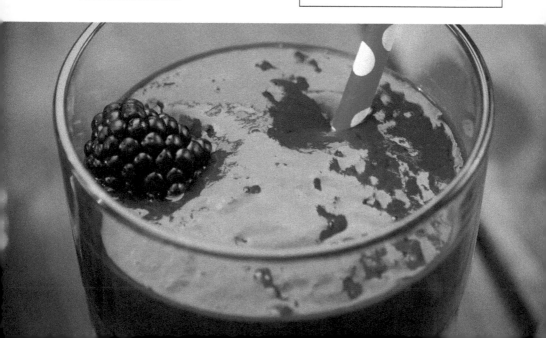

GREEN LEMONADE

INGREDIENTS

1 large bunch parsley

4 cups filtered water

stevia to taste

lemon juice to taste

Place all ingredients in a high-powered blender, and blend until uniform. Serve chilled.

Serves 3.

Recipe Tidbit:

I suggest making this beverage 2 times per week and drinking about ⅓ of it daily. I have been suggesting this blend to my patients for over a decade with excellent results. Parsley can act as a powerful blood cleanser; it also supports digestion. It is a top source of antioxidants and other nutrients, including potassium, calcium, manganese, iron, magnesium, vitamin A, beta-carotene, vitamin C, vitamin E, zeaxanthin, lutein, cryptoxanthin, and vitamin K. Fresh herb leaves such as parsley are also rich in the B vitamins, including folic acid (vitamin B9), pantothenic acid (B5), riboflavin (B2), niacin (B3), pyridoxine (B6), and thiamin (B1).

Macronutrients

Kilocalories	7.296	kcal
Trans Fatty Acid		g
Sugar, Total		g
Protein	0.602	g
Carbohydrate	2.283	g
Fat, Total	0.160	g
Alcohol	0.000	g
Cholesterol	0.000	mg
Saturated Fat	0.027	g
Monounsaturated Fat	0.060	g
Polyunsaturated Fat	0.025	g
Trans Fatty Acid	0.000	g
Dietary Fiber, Total	0.669	g
Sugar, Total	0.172	g

Percentage of Kcals

Protein	18.5%
Carbohydrate	70.3%
Fat, total	11.1%
Alcohol	0.0%

Vitamins & Minerals

Sodium	20.829	mg
Potassium	115.437	mg
Vitamin A (RE)	170.725	RE
Vitamin C	26.955	mg
Calcium	37.448	mg
Iron	1.257	mg
Vitamin D (ug)	0.000	µg
Vitamin E (mg)	0.000	mg
Thiamin	0.017	mg
Riboflavin	0.020	mg
Niacin	0.266	mg
Pyridoxine (Vitamin B6)	0.018	mg
Folate (Total)	30.805	µg
Cobalamin (Vitamin B12)	0.000	µg
Pantothenic Acid	0.081	mg
Vitamin K	332.373	µg
Phosphorus	11.755	mg
Magnesium	13.293	mg
Zinc	0.217	mg
Copper	0.058	mg
Manganese	0.032	mg
Selenium	0.020	µg

HOMEMADE ALMOND MILK

INGREDIENTS

1 cup organic whole almonds,
blanched, skins removed (see
below)

1 cup hot water

3 cups room-temperature water

Blanch almonds by boiling them in water for 1–2 minutes. Then drain, cool, and pinch off the skins.

Blend almonds with hot water in a blender until very smooth. Add remaining 3 cups water, and process until very smooth. Strain through cheesecloth into a glass container. Refrigerate.

Yields 4½ cups (9 ½-cup servings).

Recipe Tidbit:

You can try this recipe with various seeds, soybeans, or other nuts. Nuts with skins, such as Brazil nuts and hazelnuts, should be blanched and skins removed. Cashews can be used with no blanching. Some recipes call for soaking the almonds overnight, but making almond milk on the fly is possible when you blanch them. So easy! You can add vanilla extract or a mild sweetener if desired.

Making your own nut milks saves a lot of money. I don't always make my own, but I love knowing how to do so. I usually have nuts or seeds in my refrigerator that I can use in a pinch to make milk. For certain

Macronutrients		
Kilocalories	106.938	kcal
Trans Fatty Acid		g
Sugar, Total		g
Protein	3.879	g
Carbohydrate	3.384	g
Fat, Total	9.519	g
Alcohol	0.000	g
Cholesterol	0.000	mg
Saturated Fat	0.716	g
Monounsaturated Fat	6.056	g
Polyunsaturated Fat	2.242	g
Trans Fatty Acid	0.003	g
Dietary Fiber, Total	1.794	g
Sugar, Total	0.839	g

Percentage of Kcals	
Protein	13.5%
Carbohydrate	11.8%
Fat, total	74.7%
Alcohol	0.0%

Vitamins & Minerals		
Sodium	3.444	mg
Potassium	119.444	mg
Vitamin A (RE)	0.127	RE
Vitamin C	0.000	mg
Calcium	42.775	mg
Iron	0.595	mg
Vitamin D (ug)	0.000	µg
Thiamin	0.035	mg
Riboflavin	0.129	mg
Niacin	0.634	mg
Pyridoxine (Vitamin B6)	0.021	mg
Folate (Total)	8.881	µg
Cobalamin (Vitamin B12)	0.000	µg
Pantothenic Acid	0.057	mg
Vitamin K	0.000	µg
Phosphorus	87.181	mg
Magnesium	48.575	mg
Zinc	0.538	mg
Copper	0.186	mg
Manganese	0.333	mg
Selenium	0.580	µg

recipes, such as tapioca pudding, I prefer making the milk myself because I feel that fresh milk makes a much better tasting product. Same thing with flours: if a recipe calls for flour, I always have grains on hand that I can grind into a fine flour. You can do this easily in a dedicated coffee grinder, in a specialized spice grinder, or in a high-powdered blender or food processor.

TURMERIC MILK

INGREDIENTS

2 cups unsweetened almond milk

½ teaspoon powdered turmeric

pinch ground cardamom

pinch powdered ginger

pinch powdered cloves

pinch allspice

½ teaspoon vanilla extract

stevia (optional)

Combine all spices together in a bowl. Heat milk in a small saucepan, and add combined spices while stirring. Heat on low for 3–5 minutes to allow flavors to mingle. If you are using stevia, add before serving. Pour mixture through cheesecloth or tea strainer, and serve warm.

Serves 2.

Macronutrients		
Kilocalories	94.740	kcal
Trans Fatty Acid		g
Sugar, Total		g
Protein	9.054	g
Carbohydrate	5.502	g
Fat, Total	4.519	g
Alcohol	0.361	g
Cholesterol	0.000	mg
Saturated Fat	0.510	g
Monounsaturated Fat	1.003	g
Polyunsaturated Fat	2.504	g
Trans Fatty Acid	0.000	g
Dietary Fiber, Total	4.125	g
Sugar, Total	1.150	g

Percentage of Kcals	
Protein	35.7%
Carbohydrate	21.7%
Fat, total	40.1%
Alcohol	2.5%

Vitamins & Minerals		
Sodium	30.243	mg
Potassium	312.994	mg
Vitamin A (RE)	0.000	RE
Vitamin C	0.004	mg
Calcium	41.622	mg
Iron	2.130	mg
Vitamin D (ug)	0.000	µg
Thiamin	0.000	mg
Riboflavin	0.002	mg
Niacin	0.012	mg
Pyridoxine (Vitamin B6)	0.001	mg
Folate (Total)	0.110	µg
Cobalamin (Vitamin B12)	0.000	µg
Pantothenic Acid	0.003	mg
Vitamin K	0.074	µg
Phosphorus	1.708	mg
Magnesium	1.270	mg
Zinc	0.026	mg
Copper	0.008	mg
Manganese	0.111	mg
Selenium	0.034	µg

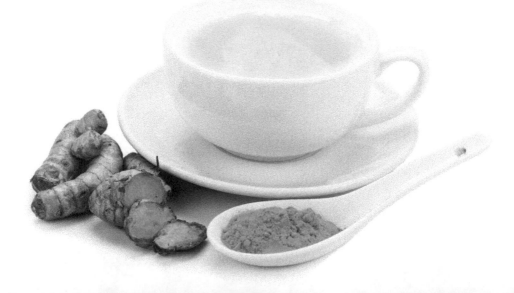

Recipe Tidbit:

Turmeric has great anti-inflammatory and healing properties. Warming the turmeric brings out its medicinal effects. This beverage could be consumed daily for improved digestive health and reduced inflammation. Reducing inflammation helps to reduce risk for cardiovascular disease, the world's number-one fatal illness.

Drinking warm milk before bed may help you sleep better. For a bedtime variation, whisk in 1 tablespoon of organic butter to help stabilize blood sugar levels throughout the night. Stabilized blood sugar will prevent hypoglycemia, which can force you awake in the middle of the night.

The next five recipes are adapted from Living with Crohn's and Colitis, which I coauthored with Dede Cummings. [Reprinted with permission of Hatherleigh Press.]

CALMING TEA

INGREDIENTS

1 part St. John's wort (St. John's wort should not be used by people taking antidepressant medication)

1 part lemon balm

1 part passionflower

Steep 1 tablespoon herb blend per 10 ounces of water. Bring appropriate amount of water to boil, remove from heat, stir in dry herbs, cover, and allow to steep for 15 minutes. Strain through fine tea strainer, cheesecloth, or clean T-shirt. Drink 3 cups daily. You can make up to 90 ounces at once and sweeten with honey if desired. If you are making bigger batches it is perfectly okay to store in the refrigerator and drink chilled.

Macronutrients

Kilocalories	2.960	kcal
Trans Fatty Acid		g
Sugar, Total		g
Protein	0.000	g
Carbohydrate	0.592	g
Fat, Total	0.000	g
Alcohol	0.000	g
Cholesterol	0.000	mg
Saturated Fat	0.006	g
Monounsaturated Fat	0.003	g
Polyunsaturated Fat	0.015	g
Dietary Fiber, Total	0.000	g
Sugar, Total	0.000	g

Percentage of Kcals

Protein	0.0%
Carbohydrate	100.0%
Fat, total	0.0%
Alcohol	0.0%

Vitamins & Minerals

Sodium	2.960	mg
Potassium	26.640	mg
Vitamin A (RE)	0.000	RE
Vitamin C	0.000	mg
Calcium	5.920	mg
Iron	0.237	mg
Vitamin D (ug)	0.000	µg
Thiamin	0.030	mg
Riboflavin	0.012	mg
Niacin	0.000	mg
Pyridoxine (Vitamin B6)	0.000	mg
Folate (Total)	2.960	µg
Cobalamin (Vitamin B12)	0.000	µg
Pantothenic Acid	0.033	mg
Vitamin K	0.000	µg
Phosphorus	0.000	mg
Magnesium	2.960	mg
Zinc	0.118	mg
Copper	0.044	mg
Manganese	0.130	mg
Selenium	0.000	µg

DETOXIFICATION AND SOOTHING TEA

INGREDIENTS

1 part licorice root

1 part marshmallow root

1 part burdock root

1 part dandelion root

1 part yellow dock root*

Yellow dock should not be used by people taking drugs that decrease blood calcium, such as diuretics, Dilantin, Miacalcin, or Mithracin. It also should not be used by people with kidney disease, liver disease, or an electrolyte abnormality.

Because these herbs are roots, the tea needs to be boiled to maximize their medicinal qualities. Add 1 tablespoon of the root mixture to 10 ounces of water. Bring to a boil, and boil for 10 minutes. Remove from heat, cover, and allow to sit for 15 minutes. Strain. Drink 3 cups daily. You can make up to 90 ounces at once and sweeten with honey if desired. If you are making bigger batches it is perfectly okay to store in the refrigerator and drink chilled.

Macronutrients		
Kilocalories	7.513	kcal
Trans Fatty Acid		g
Sugar, Total		g
Protein	0.313	g
Carbohydrate	1.223	g
Fat, Total	0.095	g
Alcohol	0.000	g
Cholesterol	0.000	mg
Saturated Fat	0.001	g
Monounsaturated Fat	0.001	g
Polyunsaturated Fat	0.005	g
Trans Fatty Acid	0.000	g
Dietary Fiber, Total	0.495	g
Sugar, Total	0.281	g

Percentage of Kcals	
Protein	17.9%
Carbohydrate	69.9%
Fat, total	12.2%
Alcohol	0.0%

Vitamins & Minerals		
Sodium	11.014	mg
Potassium	39.590	mg
Vitamin A (RE)	11.561	RE
Vitamin C	1.899	mg
Calcium	11.864	mg
Iron	0.119	mg
Vitamin D (ug)	0.000	µg
Thiamin	0.005	mg
Riboflavin	0.006	mg
Niacin	0.062	mg
Pyridoxine (Vitamin B6)	0.011	mg
Folate (Total)	5.273	µg
Cobalamin (Vitamin B12)	0.000	µg
Pantothenic Acid	0.014	mg
Vitamin K	0.045	µg
Phosphorus	8.958	mg
Magnesium	7.272	mg
Zinc	0.026	mg
Copper	0.033	mg
Manganese	0.036	mg
Selenium	0.045	µg

INFLAMMATION AND IMMUNITY TEA

INGREDIENTS

1 part pau d'arco

1 part cat's claw

1 part fresh ginger, grated fine

1 part chaparral

Steep 1 tablespoon of the mixture per 14 ounces of water. Bring appropriate amount of water to boil, remove from heat, add dry herbs, cover, and allow to steep for 15 minutes. Strain through fine tea strainer, cheesecloth, or clean T-shirt. Drink 3 cups daily. You can make up to 90 ounces at once and sweeten with honey if desired. If you are making bigger batches it is perfectly okay to store in the refrigerator and drink chilled.

Macronutrients

Kilocalories	5.103	kcal
Trans Fatty Acid		g
Sugar, Total		g
Protein	0.052	g
Carbohydrate	0.504	g
Fat, Total	0.021	g
Alcohol	0.000	g
Cholesterol	0.000	mg
Saturated Fat	0.006	g
Monounsaturated Fat	0.004	g
Polyunsaturated Fat	0.004	g
Dietary Fiber, Total	0.057	g
Sugar, Total	0.048	g

Percentage of Kcals

Protein	8.6%
Carbohydrate	83.5%
Fat, total	7.9%
Alcohol	0.0%

Vitamins & Minerals

Sodium	0.369	mg
Potassium	37.280	mg
Vitamin A (RE)	0.000	RE
Vitamin C	0.142	mg
Calcium	6.123	mg
Iron	0.301	mg
Vitamin D (ug)	0.000	µg
Thiamin	0.029	mg
Riboflavin	0.001	mg
Niacin	0.021	mg
Pyridoxine (Vitamin B6)	0.005	mg
Folate (Total)	3.147	µg
Cobalamin (Vitamin B12)	0.000	µg
Biotin	0.000	µg
Pantothenic Acid	0.034	mg
Vitamin K	0.003	µg
Phosphorus	0.964	mg
Magnesium	4.054	mg
Zinc	0.010	mg
Copper	0.063	mg
Manganese	0.120	mg
Selenium	0.020	µg

TUMMY-SOOTHING TEA

INGREDIENTS

peppermint (Should not be used in people with heartburn or reflux)

chamomile

Steep 1 tablespoon herb blend per 10 ounces of water. Bring appropriate amount of water to boil, remove from heat, add dry herbs, cover, and allow to steep for 15 minutes. Strain through fine tea strainer, cheesecloth, or clean T-shirt. Drink 3 cups daily. You can make up to 90 ounces at once. If you are making bigger batches it is perfectly okay to store in the refrigerator and drink chilled.

Macronutrients		
Kilocalories	4.819	kcal
Trans Fatty Acid		g
Sugar, Total		g
Protein	0.106	g
Carbohydrate	0.989	g
Fat, Total	0.027	g
Alcohol	0.000	g
Cholesterol	0.000	mg
Saturated Fat	0.007	g
Monounsaturated Fat	0.001	g
Polyunsaturated Fat	0.014	g
Trans Fatty Acid	0.000	g
Dietary Fiber, Total	0.227	g
Sugar, Total	0.000	g

Percentage of Kcals	
Protein	9.2%
Carbohydrate	85.6%
Fat, total	5.2%
Alcohol	0.0%

Vitamins & Minerals		
Sodium	3.714	mg
Potassium	41.645	mg
Vitamin A (RE)	12.042	RE
Vitamin C	0.902	mg
Calcium	12.559	mg
Iron	0.371	mg
Vitamin D (ug)	0.000	µg
Thiamin	0.031	mg
Riboflavin	0.019	mg
Niacin	0.048	mg
Pyridoxine (Vitamin B6)	0.004	mg
Folate (Total)	6.067	µg
Cobalamin (Vitamin B12)	0.000	µg
Pantothenic Acid	0.041	mg
Vitamin K	0.000	µg
Phosphorus	2.070	mg
Magnesium	5.103	mg
Zinc	0.145	mg
Copper	0.052	mg
Manganese	0.158	mg
Selenium	0.000	µg

GAS RELIEF TEA

INGREDIENTS

1 part fennel seeds, lightly ground
(see below)

1 part fenugreek seeds, lightly
ground

1 part althea (marshmallow) root

1 part slippery elm bark, ground
or broken apart

Use a dedicated coffee grinder or a spice grinder to grind the seeds/bark. Because these herbs are roots, seeds, and barks, the tea needs to be boiled to release their maximum medicinal qualities. Add 1 tablespoon of the mixture to 10 ounces of water. Bring water with herbs to a boil and boil for 5–10 minutes; remove from heat, cover, and allow to sit for 15 minutes. Strain and drink 3 cups daily. You can make up to 90 ounces at once and sweeten with honey if desired. If you are making bigger batches it is perfectly okay to store in the refrigerator and drink chilled.

Macronutrients		
Kilocalories	28.435	kcal
Trans Fatty Acid		g
Sugar, Total		g
Protein	1.605	g
Carbohydrate	3.777	g
Fat, Total	1.238	g
Cholesterol	0.000	mg
Saturated Fat	0.055	g
Monounsaturated Fat	0.281	g
Polyunsaturated Fat	0.048	g
Dietary Fiber, Total	1.826	g
Percentage of Kcals		
Protein	19.6%	
Carbohydrate	46.2%	
Fat, total	34.1%	
Alcohol	0.0%	
Vitamins & Minerals		
Sodium	80.938	mg
Potassium	194.591	mg
Vitamin A (RE)	0.689	RE
Vitamin C	0.992	mg
Calcium	53.070	mg
Iron	1.561	mg
Vitamin D (ug)	0.000	µg
Thiamin	0.024	mg
Riboflavin	0.022	mg
Niacin	0.255	mg
Pyridoxine (Vitamin B6)	0.030	mg
Folate (Total)	1.616	µg
Cobalamin (Vitamin B12)	0.000	µg
Phosphorus	24.097	mg
Magnesium	16.329	mg
Zinc	0.318	mg
Copper	0.082	mg
Manganese	0.231	mg
Selenium	0.179	µg

HIBISCUS TEA

INGREDIENTS

1 part chamomile flowers

1 part mint

2 parts hibiscus

Steep 1 tablespoon herb blend per 10 ounces of water. Bring appropriate amount of water to boil, remove from heat, add dry herbs, cover, and allow to steep for 15 minutes. Strain through fine tea strainer, cheesecloth, or clean T-shirt. You can make up to 90 ounces at once, store in the refrigerator, and drink chilled. Add a splash of fresh lemon juice for more tartness. I love drinking this fruity-tasting tea in place of juice because it is a beautiful red color.

Macronutrients		
Kilocalories	7.613	kcal
Trans Fatty Acid		g
Sugar, Total		g
Protein	0.170	g
Carbohydrate	1.549	g
Fat, Total	0.123	g
Alcohol	0.000	g
Cholesterol	0.000	mg
Saturated Fat	0.047	g
Monounsaturated Fat	0.013	g
Polyunsaturated Fat	0.020	g
Trans Fatty Acid	0.000	g
Dietary Fiber, Total	0.271	g
Sugar, Total	0.889	g

Percentage of Kcals	
Protein	8.5%
Carbohydrate	77.6%
Fat, total	13.9%
Alcohol	0.0%

Vitamins & Minerals		
Sodium	1.471	mg
Potassium	18.797	mg
Vitamin A (RE)	16.426	RE
Vitamin C	3.627	mg
Calcium	7.333	mg
Iron	1.436	mg
Vitamin D (ug)	0.000	µg
Thiamin	0.193	mg
Riboflavin	0.023	mg
Niacin	0.048	mg
Pyridoxine (Vitamin B6)	0.004	mg
Folate (Total)	3.528	µg
Cobalamin (Vitamin B12)	0.000	µg
Pantothenic Acid	0.011	mg
Vitamin K	0.000	µg
Phosphorus	2.514	mg
Magnesium	2.564	mg
Zinc	0.055	mg
Copper	0.022	mg
Manganese	0.040	mg
Selenium	0.000	µg

SUGAR–BALANCE TEA

INGREDIENTS

1 part green tea leaves

1 part mulberry leaves

You can purchase bulk mulberry leaves for tea from Amazon or at another website. Loose green tea leaves are easy to find in stores with a tea section. Steep 1 tablespoon herb blend per 10 ounces of water. Bring appropriate amount of water to boil, remove from heat, add dry herbs, cover, and allow to steep for 15 minutes. Strain through fine tea strainer, cheesecloth, or clean T-shirt. For an easier version, use one green tea bag with one mulberry tea bag, and double the amount of water.

Macronutrients

Kilocalories	0.652	kcal
Trans Fatty Acid		g
Sugar, Total		g
Protein	0.353	g
Carbohydrate	0.114	g
Fat, Total	0.009	g
Alcohol	0.000	g
Cholesterol	0.000	mg
Saturated Fat	0.003	g
Monounsaturated Fat	0.002	g
Polyunsaturated Fat	0.004	g
Sugar, Total	0.054	g

Percentage of Kcals

Protein	72.3%
Carbohydrate	23.3%
Fat, total	4.3%
Alcohol	0.0%

Vitamins & Minerals

Sodium	3.402	mg
Potassium	74.021	mg
Vitamin A (RE)	8.270	RE
Vitamin C	9.732	mg
Calcium	11.765	mg
Iron	0.349	mg
Vitamin D (ug)	0.000	µg
Thiamin	0.001	mg
Riboflavin	0.061	mg
Niacin	0.302	mg
Pyridoxine (Vitamin B6)	0.005	mg
Folate (Total)	2.410	µg
Cobalamin (Vitamin B12)	0.000	µg
Pantothenic Acid	0.002	mg
Vitamin K	32.318	µg
Phosphorus	4.252	mg
Magnesium	1.559	mg
Zinc	0.026	mg
Copper	0.005	mg
Manganese	0.025	mg
Selenium	0.026	µg

Chapter 7
DESSERTS

CHOCOLATE SEED BARK

INGREDIENTS

1 cup strawberries, white centers removed

140 grams organic raw cocoa butter (about 5 ounces; see below)

1 cup pumpkin seeds

1 cup sunflower seeds

⅔ cup sesame seeds

½ cup flaxseeds

½ cup chia seeds

⅓ cup organic unsweetened cocoa powder

pinch salt

Macronutrients		
Kilocalories	546.073	kcal
Trans Fatty Acid		g
Sugar, Total		g
Protein	15.666	g
Carbohydrate	19.870	g
Fat, Total	48.580	g
Alcohol	0.000	g
Cholesterol	0.525	mg
Saturated Fat	14.435	g
Monounsaturated Fat	14.546	g
Polyunsaturated Fat	13.533	g
Trans Fatty Acid	0.026	g
Dietary Fiber, Total	12.209	g
Sugar, Total	1.692	g
Percentage of Kcals		
Protein	10.8%	
Carbohydrate	13.7%	
Fat, total	75.5%	
Alcohol	0.0%	
Vitamins & Minerals		
Sodium	10.117	mg
Potassium	437.434	mg
Vitamin A (RE)	1.883	RE
Vitamin C	11.334	mg
Calcium	240.229	mg
Iron	5.966	mg
Vitamin D (ug)	0.000	µg
Vitamin E (mg)	0.184	mg
Thiamin	0.481	mg
Riboflavin	0.151	mg
Niacin	3.989	mg
Pyridoxine (Vitamin B6)	0.448	mg
Folate (Total)	73.188	µg
Cobalamin (Vitamin B12)	0.000	µg
Biotin	0.198	µg
Pantothenic Acid	0.461	mg
Vitamin K	1.745	µg
Phosphorus	529.104	mg
Magnesium	258.641	mg
Zinc	3.934	mg
Copper	1.288	mg
Manganese	1.789	mg
Selenium	21.743	µg
Molybdenum	2.416	µg

Because cocoa butter is sold in its solid form, it is best to measure it by weight. Use a kitchen scale to weigh out the proper quantity.

Puree strawberries in a food processor or blender. Melt the cocoa butter in a saucepan over low heat. Combine all ingredients in a large bowl, and pour evenly into two 10 x 15–inch baking pans that have been lined with parchment paper. Place in the freezer for about an hour. Remove from freezer, and slice the bark into 1- to 2-inch squares. Transfer to airtight containers, and store in freezer or refrigerator.

Recipe Tidbit:

You can order the raw cocoa butter online. Unsweetened cocoa powder is not a carbohydrate and therefore does not spike blood sugar levels.

This chocolate bark will be very dark. You may at first notice the absence of added sugar, but the strawberries provide just enough sweetness to make this a delicious alternative to the typical sugar-loaded chocolate. I like to store chocolate bark in the freezer so I can make big batches and not worry about its going bad before being consumed.

CAROB AVOCADO PUDDING

INGREDIENTS

2 ripe avocados

1 cup lucuma powder (see Recipe
Tidbit)

½ cup unsweetened carob powder

⅓ cup full-fat organic coconut milk

1 teaspoon vanilla extract

¼ teaspoon cinnamon

pinch salt

Remove the pits from the avocadoes, and set the pits aside. Blend all ingredients together until smooth and transfer to a medium serving bowl. Stick both avocado pits into the pudding, cover with an airtight lid or plastic wrap, and transfer to refrigerator to chill before serving. Chill for at least 1 hour.

Serves 4.

Macronutrients		
Kilocalories	427.723	kcal
Trans Fatty Acid		g
Sugar, Total		g
Protein	6.338	g
Carbohydrate	25.884	g
Fat, Total	15.150	g
Alcohol	0.361	g
Cholesterol	0.000	mg
Saturated Fat	5.657	g
Monounsaturated Fat	6.779	g
Polyunsaturated Fat	1.294	g
Trans Fatty Acid	0.000	g
Dietary Fiber, Total	10.155	g
Sugar, Total	14.663	g
Percentage of Kcals		
Protein	9.5%	
Carbohydrate	38.7%	
Fat, total	50.9%	
Alcohol	0.9%	
Vitamins & Minerals		
Sodium	32.796	mg
Potassium	499.460	mg
Vitamin A (RE)	9.867	RE
Vitamin C	6.473	mg
Calcium	57.986	mg
Iron	2.555	mg
Vitamin D (ug)	0.000	µg
Thiamin	0.061	mg
Riboflavin	0.157	mg
Niacin	1.678	mg
Pyridoxine (Vitamin B6)	0.245	mg
Folate (Total)	66.406	µg
Cobalamin (Vitamin B12)	0.000	µg
Pantothenic Acid	1.015	mg
Vitamin K	14.101	µg
Phosphorus	66.341	mg
Magnesium	33.901	mg
Zinc	0.710	mg
Copper	0.242	mg
Manganese	0.310	mg
Selenium	2.189	µg

Recipe Tidbit:

Lucuma powder is an alternative sweetener made from the dried fruit of a tree that is native to subtropical South America. It can be purchased online. It has a low glycemic index and is a good source of antioxidants and of the minerals potassium, calcium, magnesium, and phosphorus.

If you want to make this pudding without the lucuma powder, also omit the coconut milk so the pudding won't be too thin. Without the lucuma powder the pudding will be bitter, but the bitterness significantly helps with sugar cravings. It works well to substitute unsweetened cocoa powder for the carob.

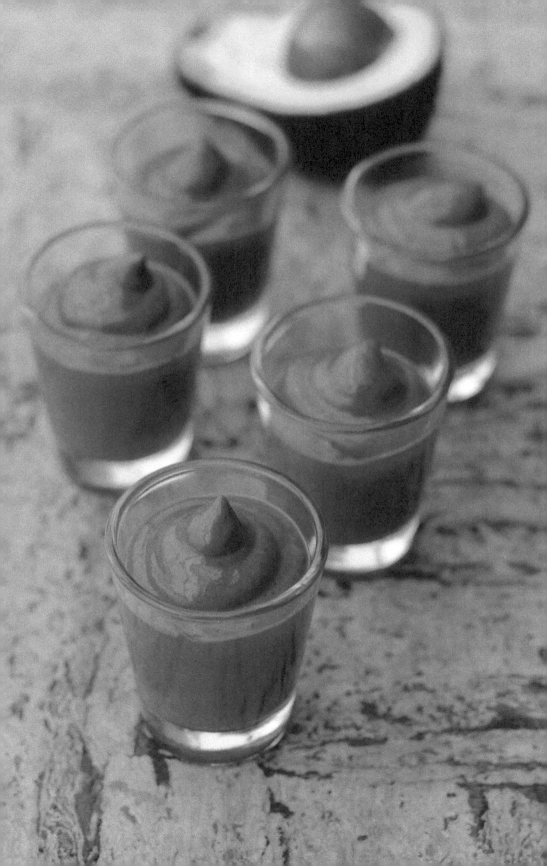

CHOCOLATE BUTTER NIBS

INGREDIENTS

1 stick unsalted butter

½ cup unsweetened sunflower
  butter

2 tablespoons unsweetened cocoa
  powder

½ cup lucuma powder (see Recipe
  Tidbit on page 184)

Melt the butter in a medium saucepan over low heat. Add sunflower
butter, and heat until softened. Stir
in cocoa powder until clumps dis-
solve, keeping the heat very low to
avoid burning. Using an inversion
blender can speed up this process.
Add the lucuma powder, and continue blending until smooth.

Macronutrients		
Kilocalories	254.742	kcal
Trans Fatty Acid		g
Sugar, Total		g
Protein	5.883	g
Carbohydrate	6.643	g
Fat, Total	17.703	g
Alcohol	0.000	g
Cholesterol	30.530	mg
Saturated Fat	8.153	g
Monounsaturated Fat	3.046	g
Polyunsaturated Fat	0.438	g
Trans Fatty Acid	0.465	g
Dietary Fiber, Total	2.448	g
Sugar, Total	2.135	g

Percentage of Kcals	
Protein	11.2%
Carbohydrate	12.7%
Fat, total	76.1%
Alcohol	0.0%

Vitamins & Minerals		
Sodium	39.333	mg
Potassium	23.982	mg
Vitamin A (RE)	106.468	RE
Vitamin C	0.000	mg
Calcium	5.136	mg
Iron	1.269	mg
Vitamin D (ug)	0.213	µg
Vitamin E (mg)	2.014	mg
Thiamin	0.002	mg
Riboflavin	0.008	mg
Niacin	0.035	mg
Pyridoxine (Vitamin B6)	0.002	mg
Folate (Total)	0.858	µg
Cobalamin (Vitamin B12)	0.024	µg
Pantothenic Acid	0.016	mg
Vitamin K	1.028	µg
Phosphorus	13.317	mg
Magnesium	57.021	mg
Zinc	0.105	mg
Copper	0.053	mg
Manganese	0.001	mg
Selenium	0.335	µg
Chromium	0.003	mg

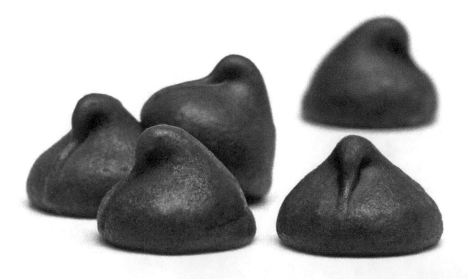

Remove from heat and set aside to cool slightly. When cool enough to handle but still liquid, transfer mixture into a gallon ziplock bag, and allow to cool until mixture is stiffer but still workable. Line 2 or 3 large baking pans with parchment paper. Cut a very small tip off the ziplock bag, and squeeze the chocolate mixture out of the bag onto the pans in ½-inch "nibs." If the mixture is still too liquid and is pouring out of the bag, clamp the cut opening, and allow to cool a little longer.

Transfer the baking sheets to the freezer, and freeze for at least 1 hour. Transfer the nibs from the baking sheets to airtight containers, and store in the freezer.

Recipe Tidbit:

When you are craving sweets, eating one or two of these can help curb those cravings. Eat no more than two, then set a timer for 5 or 10 minutes before allowing yourself to grab one or two more. The timer trick helps to keep you from bingeing on these little treats.

BAKED PEACHES WITH CINNAMON

INGREDIENTS

4 peaches, pits removed and halved

1 tablespoon vanilla extract

2 teaspoons cinnamon

1 teaspoon fresh lemon juice

¼ teaspoon salt

4 tablespoons unsalted butter

Preheat oven to 375 degrees. Place peaches in a bowl with vanilla extract, cinnamon, lemon juice, and salt, and stir until peaches are evenly coated. Arrange peaches cut side up in a baking pan. Place ½ tablespoon butter in each peach cavity. Bake for 35–45 minutes until the flesh is soft and the tops are brown.

Serves 8.

Macronutrients		
Kilocalories	172.506	kcal
Trans Fatty Acid		g
Sugar, Total		g
Protein	1.538	g
Carbohydrate	15.731	g
Fat, Total	11.912	g
Alcohol	1.084	g
Cholesterol	30.530	mg
Saturated Fat	7.328	g
Monounsaturated Fat	3.089	g
Polyunsaturated Fat	0.562	g
Trans Fatty Acid	0.465	g
Dietary Fiber, Total	2.864	g
Sugar, Total	13.049	g
Percentage of Kcals		
Protein	3.3%	
Carbohydrate	34.2%	
Fat, total	58.3%	
Alcohol	4.1%	
Vitamins & Minerals		
Sodium	147.316	mg
Potassium	299.365	mg
Vitamin A (RE)	155.715	RE
Vitamin C	10.436	mg
Calcium	24.444	mg
Iron	0.480	mg
Vitamin D (ug)	0.213	µg
Thiamin	0.038	mg
Riboflavin	0.055	mg
Niacin	1.245	mg
Pyridoxine (Vitamin B6)	0.041	mg
Folate (Total)	6.749	µg
Cobalamin (Vitamin B12)	0.024	µg
Biotin	3.000	µg
Pantothenic Acid	0.252	mg
Vitamin K	5.253	µg
Phosphorus	34.435	mg
Magnesium	14.932	mg
Zinc	0.293	mg
Copper	0.111	mg
Manganese	0.301	mg
Selenium	0.329	µg
Chromium	0.005	mg

Recipe Tidbit:

These are a deliciously sweet treat for folks who have been strictly avoiding sugar. Make sure that you balance fruit consumption with a healthy dinner containing a lot of vegetables.

DARK CHOCOLATE COCONUT BARK WITH SEA SALT

INGREDIENTS

220 grams organic raw cocoa
butter (or about 7.85 ounces; see
note on page 183)

2 cups ground unsweetened
coconut

½ cup organic cacao powder or
organic cocoa powder

½ teaspoon sea salt

Melt the cocoa butter in a saucepan over low heat. Combine with remaining ingredients, and pour contents into a parchment paper–lined 10 x 15–inch baking pan. Place in the freezer for about an hour. Remove from freezer, and slice the bark into 1- to 2-inch squares. Transfer to airtight containers, and store in freezer or refrigerator.

Macronutrients		
Kilocalories	358.712	kcal
Trans Fatty Acid		g
Sugar, Total		g
Protein	2.058	g
Carbohydrate	7.127	g
Fat, Total	38.103	g
Alcohol	0.000	g
Cholesterol	0.825	mg
Saturated Fat	25.660	g
Monounsaturated Fat	9.266	g
Polyunsaturated Fat	0.932	g
Trans Fatty Acid	0.000	g
Dietary Fiber, Total	3.793	g
Sugar, Total	1.094	g

Percentage of Kcals	
Protein	2.2%
Carbohydrate	7.5%
Fat, total	90.3%
Alcohol	0.0%

Vitamins & Minerals		
Sodium	152.272	mg
Potassium	82.296	mg
Vitamin A (RE)	0.000	RE
Vitamin C	0.000	mg
Calcium	7.250	mg
Iron	1.108	mg
Vitamin D (ug)	0.000	µg
Vitamin E (mg)	0.289	mg
Thiamin	0.004	mg
Riboflavin	0.013	mg
Niacin	0.118	mg
Pyridoxine (Vitamin B6)	0.006	mg
Folate (Total)	1.728	µg
Cobalamin (Vitamin B12)	0.000	µg
Vitamin K	0.135	µg
Phosphorus	39.636	mg
Magnesium	26.946	mg
Zinc	0.367	mg
Copper	0.204	mg
Selenium	0.772	µg

Recipe Tidbit:

This bark is very bitter, but I find it helpful as a way to curb cravings after dinner. You are welcome to add a little stevia to the mixture for sweetness, but don't overdo it; stevia can impart an even more bitter quality.

QUICK SHERBET

My husband and I were craving dessert one night, and all we had were some blackberries that I'd recently picked and frozen. I thought I'd blend them into a sherbet, and it worked! The benefits of experimenting come through again. The recipe may seem similar to a smoothie, but it really does come out like sherbet.

INGREDIENTS

2 cups frozen organic
   strawberries (you can use
   almost any berry for this recipe)
¼ cup full-fat coconut milk
mint sprig (optional, for garnish)

Put the frozen fruit in the blender and add the coconut milk. Use just enough coconut milk to get your blender going. If necessary, use a little bit more or less than the amount listed here.

Add sweetener if desired, and blend until the mixture reaches a smooth, sherbet-like consistency. Garnish with a mint sprig, and serve immediately.

Serves 4.

Recipe Tidbit:

Get creative when serving this dish. You can hollow out a lemon and spoon the sherbet into the rind.

Macronutrients		
Kilocalories	46.798	kcal
Trans Fatty Acid		g
Sugar, Total		g
Protein	0.913	g
Carbohydrate	11.276	g
Fat, Total	0.340	g
Alcohol	0.000	g
Cholesterol	0.000	mg
Saturated Fat	0.038	g
Monounsaturated Fat	0.048	g
Polyunsaturated Fat	0.185	g
Trans Fatty Acid	0.000	g
Dietary Fiber, Total	1.766	g
Sugar, Total	5.539	g

Percentage of Kcals	
Protein	7.0%
Carbohydrate	87.0%
Fat, total	5.9%
Alcohol	0.0%

Vitamins & Minerals		
Sodium	8.460	mg
Potassium	179.158	mg
Vitamin A (RE)	4.416	RE
Vitamin C	45.524	mg
Calcium	20.179	mg
Iron	0.898	mg
Vitamin D (ug)	0.000	µg
Vitamin E (mg)	0.298	mg
Thiamin	0.030	mg
Riboflavin	0.047	mg
Niacin	0.535	mg
Pyridoxine (Vitamin B6)	0.036	mg
Folate (Total)	20.284	µg
Cobalamin (Vitamin B12)	0.000	µg
Biotin	0.313	µg
Pantothenic Acid	0.132	mg
Vitamin K	2.431	µg
Phosphorus	20.614	mg
Magnesium	14.654	mg
Zinc	0.200	mg
Copper	0.064	mg
Manganese	0.320	mg
Selenium	0.773	µg

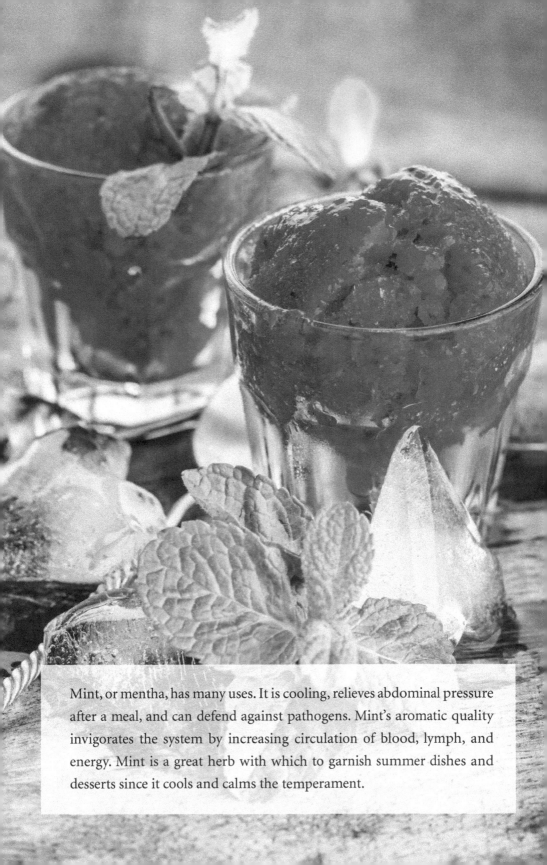

Mint, or mentha, has many uses. It is cooling, relieves abdominal pressure after a meal, and can defend against pathogens. Mint's aromatic quality invigorates the system by increasing circulation of blood, lymph, and energy. Mint is a great herb with which to garnish summer dishes and desserts since it cools and calms the temperament.

Printed in the USA
CPSIA information can be obtained
at www.ICGtesting.com
JSHW072028140824
68134JS00044B/3826